T0100276

CANCER ETIOLOGY, DIAGNOSIS AND TREATMENTS

A CONCISE HISTORY OF BREAST CANCER

CANCER ETIOLOGY, DIAGNOSIS AND TREATMENTS

Additional books in this series can be found on Nova's website under the Series tab.

Additional E-books in this series can be found on Nova's website under the E-books tab.

WOMEN'S ISSUES

Additional books in this series can be found on Nova's website under the Series tab.

Additional E-books in this series can be found on Nova's website under the E-books tab.

CANCER ETIOLOGY, DIAGNOSIS AND TREATMENTS

A CONCISE HISTORY OF BREAST CANCER

MARC LACROIX

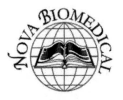

Nova Science Publishers, Inc.
New York

Library of Congress Cataloging-in-Publication Data
Lacroix, Marc, 1963-
A concise history of breast cancer / Marc Lacroix.
p. ; cm.
Includes bibliographical references and indexes.
ISBN 978-1-61122-305-7 (hardcover)
1. Breast--Cancer--History. 2. Breast--Cancer--Treatment. I. Title.
[DNLM: 1. Breast Neoplasms--history. 2. Breast Neoplasms--therapy. WP 11.1]
RC280.B8L2713 2010
616.99'449--dc22
2010035910

Published by Nova Science Publishers, Inc. †*New York*

Contents

Preface

Breast cancer is the most frequently diagnosed type of cancer and a second leading cause of cancer death in women after lung cancer. It is estimated that breast cancer affects more than 1,000,000 women worldwide each year, and about 450,000 die from the disease. During the last decades, breast cancer has received considerable attention. Yet it is a very old disease that was described millenaries ago. For long, it was observed, sometimes treated by surgery and/or traditional medicine, but rarely cured. Starting from the Renaissance, the view on the disease began to change,but significant advances in understanding and treatment of breast tumors were not achieved before the 19th century, with the notable interventions of Rudolf Virchow and William Halsted. These last 100 years have seen the explosion of knowledge on cancer and, with the notable introduction of radiotherapy, chemotherapy and endocrine therapy, the evolution towards more complex therapies. More individualized approaches (targeted therapies) are in development.

This book aims to provide a dense summary of breast cancer history. It covers the ages from the ancient times to the early 2000's, but mainly focuses on the 20th century and its numerous discoveries and inventions in the field of breast cancer detection, analysis and treatment.

The fields covered here are: surgery, radiotherapy, chemotherapy, endocrine therapy, targeted therapy, staging and grading systems, genetics, imaging and detection, and breast cancer models.

Born in 1963 inVerviers (Wallonia, Belgium), Marc Lacroix has been working for more than 20 years in several academic institutions (University of Liège, Free University of Brussels, Jules Bordet Institute). He is now at InTextoResearch (ITR@iname.com, 4 chemin de Hoevel, B-4837 Baelen, Belgium), an agency devoted to scientific information on cancer.

Chapter 1

From Prehistoric Times to the End of the Middle Ages

Abstract

Breast cancer is a very old disease. Cases described as "breast cancer" were reported in various civilizations, from Ancient Egypt to the Western Middle Ages. Tumor progression was also mentioned. It was recognized that breast cancer was among the most widespread cancers. The causes of the disease were not clearly identified. Proposed by Hippocrates and later defended by Galen, the "humoral theory", based on the imbalance of four biological humors – blood, phlegm, black bile and yellow bile, was predominant for centuries. The therapeutic armamentarium was poor and pragmatic. It included tumor excision and/or cauterization, but also the application of compounds such as arsenical pastes, herbs, oil, heavy metals....

Cancer is often seen as a contemporary disease, but is in fact very old. For instance, Kenyan paleontologist Louis *Seymour Bazett* Leakey (1903-1972) found the oldest possible hominid malignant tumor in 1932 in the so-called "Kanam Mandible", which was assigned to archaic Homo of the African Middle Pleistocene or the Late Pleistocene. The observed "exophytic mass" [Sandison 1975; Phelan *et al.* 2007] had features suggestive of a Burkitt's lymphoma. Nasopharyngeal carcinomas and osteogenic sarcomas were identified in Egyptian [Strouhal 1978] or Peruvian mummies dating back to approximately 3000-1500 BC. Lesions suggesting multiple bone metastases from carcinomas have also been described in Egyptian mummies dating from approximately 1500-500 BC, but it was impossible to conclude whether the corresponding primary tumors were breast tumors [Zink *et al.* 1999].

Egypt

Perhaps the earliest record of breast cancer is mentioned on the so-called "Edwin Smith Papyrus", written in the hieratic script of the ancient Egyptian language and discovered in Egypt in 1862. Edwin Smith (1822-1906) was an American Egyptologist. The papyrus is a sixteen-foot long roll now housed in the BritishMuseum. The document traces to about the 16th to 17th century BC but actually is the only surviving copy of part of a much older treatise on trauma surgery from about 3000 to 2500 BC. Translation of hieratic was undertaken by American archaeologist and historian James *Henry* Breasted (1865-1935), aided by American physiologist Arno *Benedict* Luckhardt (1885-1957). The text is attributed to Imhotep, the "god of healing", credited with being the founder of Egyptian medicine.It details eight cases of breast tumors (or "ulcers"). The exact nature of the diseases described in the papyrus has been intensively discussed, and it was concluded that some "tumors" could in fact be infections or abcesses (discussed in [Weiss 2000]). No treatment is proposed, except cauterization with a "fire drill", in one case. Indeed, at this time, tumors were mainly, if not uniquely, treated with cautery of the diseased tissue.

China

What is reputed as the earliest surviving medical book, the "Huang Ti Nei Ching Su Wên", or "The Yellow Emperor's Classic of Internal Medicine", presents itself as the teachings of a legendary Celestial Master addressed to Huang Ti, the Yellow Emperor (c. 2600 BC).The existence of Huang Ti is controversial, but he is venerated as the Father of Chinese Medicine. The existing text (dated c. 250 BC) is likely a reworking of an earlier version that could have been completed about five centuries before. It contains a clinical picture of breast cancer, including progression, metastasis and death. The book describes illness as imbalance between the "yang"—the active, warm, dry, light, positive, masculine principle; and the "yin"—the cold, wet, dark, negative, feminine principle, and also between the five elements (earth, fire, air, water, and metal). Treatment involves various methods to restore balance. The "Nei Ching" lists five methods of treatment, said to have been developed in historical succession: "The first method cures the spirit; the second gives knowledge on how to nourish the body; the third teaches on the true effects of medicines; the fourth explains acupuncture and the use of the small and large needle; the fifth gives instruction on how to examine and treat the bowels and the viscera, the blood, and the breath".

India

Most ancient civilizations show reference to a breast disease that could be cancer. For instance, writings from India dating back to approximately 2000 BC document the treatment methods of breast cancer as surgical excision, cautery, and arsenic compounds. In the Indian epic tale "Ramayana" ("Rama's way" in sanskrit), it is mentioned that arsenic pastes were administered as long ago as 500 BC to slow down tumor growth.

Persia

According to Herodotus (c. 484 – c. 425 BC), Democedes of Croton (c. 558 BC – c. 460 BC) was a Greek physician who was captured by the Persians and is said to have cured king Darius I of a lesion of the ankle that Egyptian doctors could not heal. Later on, Darius's wife, Atossa, had a swelling on her breast. She was cured by Democedes. It is unclear whether Atossa's disease was breast cancer. Indeed, the clinical description of the lesion, and the fact that it was apparently cured only by a simple excision followed by the application of herbs, suggests an abscess rather than a cancer (discussed in [Weiss 2000]).

Greece

The most famous of Greek physicians, Hippocrates of Cos (c. 460 BC – c. 370 BC), first used the words "carcinos" and "carcinoma", from the Greek term "karkinos", referring to a crab. Hippocrates or a Hippocratic writer compared the long, distended veins radiating from a breast tumor to the limbs of a crab. Furthermore, the word "cancer" means crab or crayfish in Latin. Hippocrates occasionally mentioned breast cancer. In one case, he tells of a woman in Abdera who developed carcinoma of the breast with bloody discharge from her nipple, and once the flow stopped, she died [Karpozilos and Pavlidis 2004]. However, this is not the usual hallmark of breast cancer, but it certainly is for breast duct papilloma, a benign condition of the breast. It has also been suggested that it could have been a case of epithelioma.

Before the Greeks, medicine was strongly influenced by religion. Hippocrates used systematic observation and logical thinking to propose the humoral theory of cancer. According to this theory, the human body contains a mixture of four biological humors—blood, phlegm, black bile, and yellow bile, which are the counterparts of the Empedocle's four cardinal elements of the universe: air, water, earth and fire, respectively. A proper balance of these four fluids results in a state of health whereas an imbalance produces disease, with cancer specifically stemming from an accumulation of excess black bile at the afflicted body site.Treatment consists in restoring balance through diet, exercise, and the judicious use of herbs, oils, earthly compounds, and occasionally heavy metals or surgery. Hippocrate's stepwise treatment approach is summarized in one of his Aphorisms. "What drugs will not cure, the knife will; what the knife will not cure, the cautery will; what the cautery will not cure must be considered incurable". For internal cancers, Hippocrates stated, "It is better not to apply any treatment in cases of a cancer; for the ones who are treated die sooner, while those who are not treated survive a longer time" [Gallucci 1985; Diamandopoulos 1996]

With the decline and fall of ancient Greece, the humoral theory of cancer passed on to the Romans and was accepted by the influential Roman physician Galen. In fact, this theory remained unchallenged for over 1,300 years. Knowledge stagnated during this extended period of time, notably because religious beliefs prohibited the study of the body, including carrying out autopsies.

Rome

Approximately four centuries after Hippocrates, Roman physician Aulus Cornelius Celsus (c. 25 BC – c. 50 AD) observed the frequent appearance of secondary tumors after the primary one had been removed. He thus admitted the distant propagation of the tumor: "After excision, even when a scar has formed, none the less the disease has returned." Celsus wrote this about breast cancer, "We have often seen in the breast a tumor exactly resembling the animal the crab. Just as the crab has legs on both sides of his body, so in this disease the veins extending out from the unnatural growth take the shape of a crab's legs. We have often cured this disease in its early stages, but after it has reached a large size no one has cured it without operation. In all operations we attempt to excise a pathological tumor in a circle in the region where it borders the healthy tissue."

Celsus was the first to operate breast cancer and to ligate blood vessels during the operation. In general, however, Celsus advised against surgery, but also against cautery, and caustic medicines. The early Romans performed extensive surgery for cancer of the breast, including removal of the pectoral muscles.Leonides of Alexandria (c. 180) was the first to describe retraction of the nipple in breast cancer. He performed mastectomy, but advised against this treatment for advanced disease [Weiss 2000]. He was more concerned about hemorrhage and he is credited of being the first to use a scalpel and cautery alternately as he proceeded around the tumor until the breast had been amputated. Cautery aimed to stem the flow of blood during and after surgery, and to destroy any residual cancer tissue.Claudius Galenus, known as Galen of Pergamum (131–203), a Greek physician, pharmacist, and philosopher, thought much as Hippocrates had. Galen came to Rome at a young age to establish his practice and became physician to the Roman Emperor Marcus Aurelius. Galen is often regarded as the founder of clinical medicine and the first oncologist. He wrote about cancers of multiple different organs, including the female reproductive tract, the intestines, and the breast.His major contribution to understanding cancer was the classification of tumors into: *tumores secondum naturam* (tumors according to nature) which included physiologic processes such as the growth of breasts during puberty or of the pregnant uterus; *tumores supra naturam* (tumors above nature), such as abscesses or inflammations; and, *tumores praeter naturam* (tumors beyond nature). He subdivided the latter into: *onkoi* (lumps or masses in general), *karkinos* (included malignant ulcers), and *karkinomas* (included non-ulcerating cancers).Galen believed extreme depression ("melancholia") to be the chief factor in the development of breast cancer, leading to a coagulum of black bile within the breast. To eliminate this excess of black bile, he prescribed treatment with topical application of various herbs, special diets, and even exorcism. Galen said that once a patient was diagnosed with cancer there was no definitive cure. However, although he cautioned, like Hippocrates did, against treatment of hidden cancers, arguing that treatment more often than not hastened death, he thought surgery could in some cases cure the cancer if the tumor was completely removed in its earliest stages. The control of hemorrhage was by the use of pressure on surrounding veins as ligatures were thought to cause local recurrence of breast cancer. The humoral theory of cancer, as defended by Hippocrates and Galen, was maintained through the Middle Ages and was substantially challenged only starting from the early 19th century.

Byzance

During the Byzantine period the most prominent medical personalities were Oribasius (c. 320-400), Aëtius of Amida (6th century) and Paul of Aegina (c. 625 – c. 695). They were most seen as compilers, or encyclopedists, rather than novators in the field of cancer, as they preserved the medical teachings of Hippocrates and Galen. They all recognized that breast cancer was among the most wide-spread cancers. For instance, Paul of Aegina wrote a seven volume "Epitome of Medicine". In his opinion, cancer of the breast and uterus were the most common. In the sixth book of the Epitome, exclusively to do with surgery, he asserted that surgery on uterine cancer was useless. For breast cancer, he recommended removal as opposed to cauterization (see [Gurunluoglu and Gurunluoglu 2003]), even for advanced tumors. The operation should be accompanied by the administration of a fortifiant regime and an invocation to Saint Agatha, a women who had been martyred in Sicily, in the 3rd century, by a Roman governor who ordered her breasts torn off with iron shears. For centuries, Constantinople (the former Byzance) was the intellectual headquarters of medicine, serving as a vital crossroads in the preservation and dispersal of medical wisdom. The ancient teachings of Hippocrates and Galen continued to inspire physicians in Constantinople, but also in Cairo, Alexandria, and Athens. During this period the cause of cancer was explained as the result of an excess of black bile.

Islamic Spain

Islamic scholars translated Greek and Roman works, spreading knowledge west to Spain and east to Persia and Baghdad. An Islamic surgeon born in

Spain (1013-1106), Abulkassim Al-Zahrawi, better known as Abulcasis or Abulcassis discussed about breast cancer and its removal.

He thought surgery should be attempted only if the tumor was small and found in an early stage. He wrote that he had never been able to cure breast cancer, nor did he know anyone who had. He believed that before surgery was performed, the patient first had to be purged of bile and possibly have her veins bled.

Middle Ages

This period was a time of superstition regarding disease treatment, including treatment for breast cancer. The power of the Roman Catholic Church was a great influence on science; because of the church's influence, people of those times believed illness was a result of sin and a punishment from God. Surgery and cautery was used on smaller tumors. Caustic pastes, usually containing arsenic, were used on more extensive cancers, as well as phlebotomy, diet, herbal medicines, and symbolic charms.The Italian physician and surgeon Guido Lanfranchi (c. 1250 – c. 1306) devoted most of his practice to diseases of the breast. He gave the first description of how to differentiate benign enlargement of the breast from cancer [Hajdu 2004].

In the late Middle Ages, Henri de Mondeville (1260-1320), the first important French surgeon, refined Galen's black bile theory. He distinguished between black bile from the liver, which caused a hard tumor in the breast (a sclerosis) and twice combusted bile derived from breakdown of blood, phlegm, and yellow bile, which caused a "true" cancer. He described true cancer as ulcerated with thick margins and having an offensive odor. Mondeville thought that no cancer may be cured, unless being radically extirpated entirely.

He thus advocated surgery only for small tumors. Curiously, Mondeville argued that laughter facilitates recovery from surgery, while negative emotions slow recovery.Breast cancer is discussed by other famous medieval surgeons, such as the French Gui de Chauliac (c. 1300-1368), often seen as the father of modern surgery, and John of Arderne (1307-1392), who notably described male breast cancer [Ravandi-Kashani and Hayes 1998].

References

Diamandopoulos GT. Cancer: an historical perspective. *Anticancer Res.* 1996 Jul-Aug;16(4A):1595-602.

Gallucci BB. Selected concepts of cancer as a disease: from the Greeks to 1900. *Oncol. Nurs. Forum.* 1985 Jul-Aug;12(4):67-71.

Gurunluoglu R, Gurunluoglu A. Paul of Aegina: landmark in surgical progress. *World J. Surg.* 2003 Jan;27(1):18-25.

Hajdu SI. Medieval pathfinders in surgical oncology. *Cancer.* 2004 Sep 1;101(5):879-82.

Karpozilos A, Pavlidis N. The treatment of cancer in Greek antiquity. *Eur. J.Cancer.* 2004 Sep;40(14):2033-40.

Phelan J, Weiner MJ, Ricci JL, J.Plummer T, Gauld S, Potts R, R. Bromage TG. Diagnosis of the Pathology of the Kanam Mandible. *Oral Surg. Oral Med. Oral Pathol. Oral Radiol. Endod.* 2007 Apr;103(4):e20.

Ravandi-Kashani F, Hayes TG. Male breast cancer: a review of the literature. *Eur. J. Cancer.* 1998 Aug;34(9):1341-7.

Sandison AT. Letter: Kanam mandible's tumour. *Lancet.* 1975 Feb 1;1(7901):279.

Strouhal E. Ancient Egyptian case of carcinoma. *Bull. N. Y. Acad. Med.* 1978 Mar;54(3):290-302.

Weiss L. Metastasis of cancer: a conceptual history from antiquity to the 1990s. *Cancer Metastasis Rev.* 2000;19(3-4):I-XI, 193-383.

Zink A, Rohrbach H, Szeimies U, Hagedorn HG, Haas CJ, Weyss C, Bachmeier B, Nerlich AG. Malignant tumors in an ancient Egyptian population. *Anticancer Res.* 1999 Sep-Oct;19(5B):4273-7.

Chapter 2

Fifteenth to Eighteenth Centuries

Abstract

Starting in the 15th century, scientists and surgeons began to better understand the human body. With Renaissance, learning and medical teaching were revived. Moreover, creativity and rebellion against dogma were rediscovered. For the first time in almost 1500 years, the "humoral theory" of the origin of cancer was challenged and new hypotheses were formulated, with a predominance of the "lymph theory". The bases of pathologic anatomy and experimental oncology were thrown. The term "metastasis" was coined to describe the invasion of bloodstream by cancer cells. Surgery for breast cancer was, however, still a risky operation at that time. Operations were long and painful, due to the lack of anesthesia and antiseptic conditions.

Physician Philippus *Theophrastus Aureolus Bombastus* von Hohenheim (1493-1541), called Paracelsus, meaning "beyond Celsus" (the early Roman physician, see Chapter 1), thought that cancer was a product of excess or deficiency of certain fluids rather than an imbalance in the body's humors. He proposed to substitute Galen's black bile by"*ens*" (entities): *ens astrorum* (cosmic influences differing with climate and country); *ens veneni* (toxic matter originating in the food); *ens naturale et spirituale* (defective physical or mental constitution); and *ens deale* (an affliction sent by Providence). He refused to accept medical teaching not based on experience (empiricism). He pioneered a natural philosophy founded on chemical principles and introduced chemicals like laudanum, sulfur, lead, and mercury in therapy.

In the field of surgery, Ambroise Paré (1510-1590) was one of the most important figures of the Renaissance. Rejected by medical schools, he was educated on the battlefields of France's armies. This allowed him to rise from the humble status of barber's apprentice to become surgeon to the kings of France. Paré used an alternative to cauterization when excising breast tumors: he mixed egg white, turpentine, and rose oil for a more effective and less painful way to seal a wound. Paré recommended surgery for cancer only if the cancer could be totally removed. However, the lack of knowledge on cancer at his time led him to declare, "Any kind of cancer is almost incurable and... (if operated)...heals with great difficulty". Paré also noted that "When (cancer) possesses the breast, it often causes inflammation to the arm holes, and send the swelling even to the glandules thereof", and that patients with axillary lymph node involvement following mastectomy had a poor prognosis [Weiss 2000].

Andreas Vesalius (1514-1564) was a professor of anatomy at Padua University in Italy, and he urged physicians to understand the human body through dissection. Because the Church prohibited dissection, he often took bodies from graves and even stole from the gallows in secret. Vesalius is seen as the founder of scientific anatomy. His book, "De Humani Corporis Fabrica" ("On the Fabric of the Human Body"), depicted the human body in greater detail than ever before recorded. He used ligatures instead of hot cautery to control bleeding after excision of breast cancers. As Vesalius failed to confirm the existence of black bile, his work contributed strongly to the rejection of the old "humoral theory" of cancer. The door was open for the related "lymph theory" (see below).

However, Gabriele Fallopio, or Falloppio (1523-1562), pupil and successor of Andreas Vesalius in Padua, still considered that a blend of blood and melancholic humors was the cause of breast cancer. He also thought that cancer could be diagnosed retrospectively by the ineffectiveness of treatment. He distinguished between benign and malignant tumors, a distinction largely applicable today. He recognized malignant tumors by their woody firmness, irregular shape, multi-lobulation, adhesion to neighboring tissues (skin, muscles, and bones), and by their surrounding congested blood vessels. In contrast, benign tumors were said to be softer masses of regular shape (often round) that are movable and do not adhere to adjacent structures. He also advocated a cautious approach to cancer treatment, "Quiescente cancro, medicum quiescentrum" ("When the cancer is quiescent, the physician should also be quiescent") [Weiss 2000]. He was the first to describe the pectoral fixation of the tumor in advanced breast cancer and used this physical sign as evidence of inoperability.

Jacques Guillemeau (1550–1613), a favored student of Ambroise Paré and a surgeon at Hôtel-Dieu de Paris, advocated removal of the pectoralis muscle along with the breast. Guillemeau succeeded Paré as surgeon to the king.

In his "Opera Observationum et Curationum Medico-Chirurgicarum Quae Extant Omnia" ("Compendium of all Medico-Surgical Observations and Treatments"), Wilhelm Fabricius Hildanus (1560-1634), also known as Fabrice of Hilden, recognized the axillary nodes involvement in breast cancer. He is considered as the "Father of German surgery » and seems to have been the first to remove enlarged lymph nodes when performing breast cancer operations.

William Harvey (1578-1657) announced the discovery of the human circulatory system in 1628, in his "Exercitatio Anatomica de Motu Cordis et Sanguinis in Animalibus", (An Anatomical Exercise on the Motion of the Heart and Blood in Living Beings) and stated that blood re-circulates in the system. This was the 17th century's most significant achievement in medicine and physiology.

Like Ambroise Paré and Fabrice of Hilden, Marcus Aurelius Severinus (1580–1656) recognized the axillary involvement in breast cancer and advocated removal of axillary lymph nodes along with the breast. In 1632, Severinus was the author of the first illustrated work on surgical pathology and comparative anatomy, "Recondita Abscessuum Natura" ("On the Obscure Nature of Abscesses"). The book, a landmark in the field, included descriptions of neoplasms and provided illustrations of cases [Reichert 1929]. Severinus described benign and malignant breast tumors and their differential diagnostic [Ekmektzoglou 2009]. He advocated the excision of benign tumors, given the risk of degeneration of this type of lesions.

Gaspare Aselli (1581-1626) discovered lymph (named "chyle", 1622) and the lymphatic vessels through experiments on animals. He inferred (incorrectly) that this liquid flowed into the liver, where he assumed that it was 'concocted' into blood, as the classical physiology taught. The description of lymphatic system, completed by the French Jean Pecquet (1622 – 1674), the Dane Thomas Bartholin (1616 – 1680) and the Swedish Olof Rudbeck (1630 – 1702) [Ambrose 2007], and the demonstration of lymph final drainage into the blood circulation (discovered by Harvey), led to the conclusion that black bile, as mentioned in the "humoral theory" of cancer, could be found nowhere, whereas lymph was everywhere.Lymph thus became highly suspect and soon replaced black bile as one of the cardinal biological liquids. This ultimately led to a theory attributing cancer to lymph abnormalities. As a consequence, lymph nodes were more frequently removed when enlarged and near the tumor site. Lymphatic drainage became the key factor in developing more extensive surgical removal of cancer.

German surgeons Johannes Scultetus (1595-1645) [Scultetus *et al.* 2003] and Lorenz (or Laurentius) Heister (1683-1758) believed removing cancers was possible and performed total mastectomies, although these surgical outcomes were often unfavorable. In addition to removing the cancerous breast with the axillary contents and the pectoralis muscle, Heister removed ribs as well if necessary, an operation still occasionally performed today for stable local disease.

In 1637, the French René Descartes (1590-1650) published his "Discours De La Méthode Pour Bien Conduire Sa Raison Et Chercher La Vérité Dans Les Sciences" ("Discourse on the Method of Rightly Conducting One's Reason and of Seeking Truth in the Sciences"). This philosophical treatise on the method of systematic doubt was pivotal in guiding thinkers and researchers in their quest for the truth. After the discovery of the lymphatic system, Descartes proposed that spontaneous coagulation of defective lymph in extravascularized blood could produce breast cancer. The concept was refined by John Hunter (1728–1793). This concept, although conceptually little better than Galen's black bile theory, may however have been a stimulus for encouraging surgeons to remove obviously affected axillary lymph nodes.

Italian physician and philosopher Bernardino Ramazzini (1633-1714), of Padua, is known as the « Father of industrial/occupational medicine », as he systematically studied the relationship between work and diseases. He observed an unusually high incidence of breast cancer among nuns. This observation was repeated by many others, and has been supported by recent research suggesting that prolonged exposure to hormonal activity because of early menarche or late menopause, or the years of reproductive life uninterrupted by pregnancies, increases the risk of genetic damage and can result in breast cancer.

Based on the recent knowledge of lymphatic and blood systems, two German physicians and chemists of Halle, Friedrich Hoffmann (1660-1740) and Georges-Ernest Stahl (1660-1734) proposed in 1695 that life consists of continuous and appropriate movement of body fluids, such as blood and lymph, through solid parts. Thus, according to Stahl, life is a purely mechanical process, or "living body is nothing else than that which has structure". The lymph theory further contended that benign tumors were caused by local coagulation of lymph leaked from lymphatic vessels, whereas malignant cancers instead arose from the fermentation and degeneration of lymph. This theory dominated medical thinking for nearly 150 years but was eventually abandoned due to a lack of confirmatory evidence.

Lumpectomy and mastectomy were performed in the 17th century by the Dutch surgeon Adrian Helvetius (circa 1661–1727), who believed surgery was a cure for cancer. In 1697, he published a "Lettre sur la Nature et la Guérison du Cancer" ("Letter on the Nature and Cure of Cancer") describing the case of Marguerite Perpointe, a forty-eight-year-old Englishwoman he had treated. He had recommended surgery the first time he examined her, but she was too scared and tried many other supposed remedies over a six-month period, while the tumor in her breast grew from the size of a walnut to the size of a fist. Finally she agreed to the surgery, which went "without great pain, without cries, without the appearance of weakness, without the slightest danger, without spilling more than two palettes of blood, with ease, facility, and promptness." All that was removed was the hardened mass, but apparently the woman's scar healed and her health went back to normal" [Gros 2008].

During the 17th century, various surgical instruments began to be developed which allowed very rapid amputation of the breast, perhaps in as little as 2 or 3 seconds. The majority of these techniques involved using metal rings or forks to transfix the breast and distract it from the chest wall, thereby allowing rapid amputation with either a knife or a hinged scythe. The large wounds thus created took months to heal and therefore these were gradually abandoned.

French monk Jean Godinot (1661-1744) recognized that the special needs of cancer patients were not being met. He opened in 1740 the first cancer hospital, in Reims (France). It initially welcomed 5 women and 3 men, in the midst of strong protestations by neighborhood inhabitants. At that time, cancer was considered to be contagious.

Rejecting the 17th-century theory that cancer was primarily caused by abnormalities in the lymph and lymphatic system, a French physician, Claude Gendron (1663-1750) suggested that cancer arises locally as a hard, growing mass, untreatable with drugs, and must be removed with all its "filaments."

Dutch physician Hermann Boerhaave (1668-1738) proposed that cancer was the most unfavorable outcome of inflammation, which in turn, was due initially to stasis of circulating humors, particularly of the lymph.

Jean-Louis Petit (1674-1750), director of the French surgical academy, is credited with developing the first unified concept for the surgical treatment of breast cancer [Kardinal and Yarbro 1979]. In his writings, published 24 years after his death, Petit suggested that "...the roots of cancer were the enlarged lymphatic glands; that the glands should be looked for and removed and that the pectoral fascia and even some fibers of the muscle itself should be dissected away rather than leave any doubtful tissue. The mammary gland too should not be cut into during the operation".

The development of pathologic anatomy was aided by the removal of bans against dissection and autopsy. Italian anatomist Giovanni Battista Morgagni (1682-1771) was the first to perform autopsies to relate the patient's illness to their pathologic findings postmortem.Cancer could now be detected, albeit after death. Morgagni, considered the "Father of modern pathology", studied about 700 cases and published his observations in 1761 in his book « De Sedibus Et Causis Morborum Per Anatomen Indagatis » ("On the Seats and Causes of Diseases as Investigated by Anatomy").

French physician Jean Astruc (1684-1766) and chemist Bernard Peyrilhe (1735-1804) illustrated the beginnings of experimental oncology. They conducted research to confirm or disprove contemporary theories related to the origin of cancer, sometimes through strange ways. For example, in 1740, Astruc sought to test the validity of the humoral theory by comparing the taste of boiled beef steak with that of boiled breast tumor; he found no black-bile-like taste in the tumor. Peyrilhe tried to demonstrate an infective cause for cancer by injecting human cancer tissue into a dog. The resultant infected abcess (no cancer!) resulted in a housemaid drowning the poor dog to end its misery.

Based on previous demonstrations of lymph and blood systems, Henri-François Le Dran (1685-1770) rejected the humoral theory of cancer. He advanced the theory that cancer began in its earliest stages as a local disease, spread first to the lymph nodes and subsequently entered the circulation [Le Dran 1757]. He advocated surgery as the only treatment of localized breast cancer, but believed that once cancer had spread through lymphatics, it was inoperable and fatal. Le Dran argued that lymph node dissections should become an integral part of the surgical management of breast cancer.

In the 17th through 19th centuries, physicians who studied breast cancer and performed mastectomy worldwide were mostly of the opinion that the entire breast should be removed (including the axillary nodes), in order to give the patient a greater chance of living a normal life. Operations were long and painful, but it seems that women with cancer frequently required surgical treatment, although it was usually too late.

During the 18th century, the antique humoral theory was progressively replaced by the lymph theory. Proposed by René Descartes, it was promoted by prominent French surgeons, including Le Dran and Antoine Louis (1723-

1792). Louis distinguished cancer types based according to the manner of lymph coagulation.

The lymph theory was perpetuated by the Scottish John Hunter (1728–1793), a major surgeon and medical scientist of the 18th century. He believed that breast cancer arose when defective lymph coagulated, and that coagulation could be a consequence of inflammation, itself viewed a healthy reaction to injury. Hunter suggested that, if tumor has not encroached to the nearby tissue and was still moveable, there was no impropriety in removing it. Hunter and his disciples advocated the removal of enlarged lymph nodes in patients with primary breast cancer.

With the acceptance of the local origin of cancer, the principles of curative surgery were to perform wide en bloc operations at the earliest moment. As early as 1773, Bernard Peyrilhe advised an operation that removed the cancerous breast with the axillary contents and the pectoralis muscle, the same operation introduced by William Halsted 100 years later.

Matthew Baillie (1761–1823) wrote the first systemic illustrated pathology textbook based on organs (1793). This book, "The Morbid Anatomy of Some of the Most Important Parts of the Human Body", is considered the first systematic study of pathology, and the first publication in English on pathology as a separate subject. Cancers of breast are described. The pioneering contributions of Morgagni (see above) and Baillie are often seen as milestones in the development of morbid anatomy.

Xavier Bichat's (1771–1802) concept of tissues, developed without the use of a microscope at the end of the 18th century, laid the groundwork for structural and pathologic anatomy. Bichat stated that each system of tissues had its own characteristic lesions. Cancer was thought to be cellular tissue. Bichat's pupil, René Laennec (1781–1826), better known as the inventor of the stethoscope than as a pathologist, made a distinction between inflammation, such as gangrene, and cancer, which was an accidental tissue. He separated inflammatory from true tumors and pointed out that disease processes were both local and general. Thus, Laennec took Bichat's tissues of the body and made them into a classification of disease [Stone *et al.* 2003].

French Joseph Récamier (1774-1852) observed the invasion of blood stream by cancer cells, coining the term metastasis (1829), which came to mean the distant spread of cancer from its primary site to other places in the body. Récamier classified cancer as unilocal or multilocal in origin; the multilocal was generalized metastatic disease, which he considered to be incurable.

In 1775, Percival Pott (1714-1788) surgically treated a young woman with "ovarian herniae," and thereafter observed that mammary development was influenced by ovariectomy [Pott 1775].

In 1836, English surgeon Astley Cooper (1768-1841) observed that advanced breast cancer appeared to wax and wane during phases of the menstrual cycle [Brock 1969].

Fanny Burney (1752-1840), a much praised novelist, playwright and writer of journals and letters, related her mastectomy performed without anesthesics by Dominique-Jean Larrey (1776–1842), Napoleon's surgeon [Epstein 1986].

References

Ambrose CT. Rudbeck's complaint: a 17th-century Latin letter relating to basic immunology. *Scand. J. Immunol.* 2007 Oct;66(4):486-93.

Brock RC. The life and work of Sir Astley Cooper. *Ann. R. Coll. Surg. Engl.* 1969 Jan;44(1):1-18.

Ekmektzoglou KA, Xanthos T, German V, Zografos GC. Breast cancer: from the earliest times through to the end of the 20th century. *Eur. J. Obstet. Gynecol. Reprod. Biol.* 2009 Jul;145(1):3-8.

Epstein JL. Writing the unspeakable: Fanny Burney's mastectomy and the fictive body. *Representations* (Berkeley). 1986;(16):131-66.

Gros D. Marguerite Perpointe, une opérée du sein en 1690 (in French). *OncoMagazine.* 2008 Aug;2(3):27-32.

Reichert FL. Marcus Aurelius Severinus (1580-1656): A Contemporary of Harvey, and Author of the First Work on Comparative Anatomy. *Cal. West Med.* 1929 Mar;30(3):183-5.

Kardinal CG, Yarbro JW. A conceptual history of cancer. *Semin. Oncol.* 1979 Dec;6(4):396-408.

LeDran HF. Memoires avec un précis de plusieurs observations sur le cancer. *Mem. Acad. R. Chir.* 1757;3:1–54

Pott P. An ovarian hernia. *The Chirurgical Works* (London).1775:791–2.

Scultetus AH, Villavicencio JL, Rich NM. The life and work of the German physician Johannes Scultetus (1595-1645). *J. Am. Coll. Surg.* 2003 Jan;196(1):130-9.

Stone MJ, Aronoff BE, Evans WP, Fay JW, Lieberman ZH, Matthews CM, Race GJ, Scruggs RP, Stringer CA Jr. History of the Baylor Charles A.

Sammons Cancer Center. Proc (Bayl Univ Med Cent). 2003 Jan;16(1):30-58.

Weiss L. Metastasis of cancer: a conceptual history from antiquity to the 1990s. Chapter 7: the morphologic documentation of clinical progression, invasion metastasis – staging. *Cancer Metastasis Rev.* 2000;19(3-4):I-XI, 193-383.

Chapter 3

Nineteenth Century

Abstract

During the 19th century, the knowledge of the causes of cancer was revolutionized, as the "cellular theory", initiated by Rudolph Virchow replaced the "lymph theory". In surgery, this new theory led to the development of radical mastectomy, with William Halsted as a major initiator. Significant progresses were made in anesthesiology and asepsy. Due to the use of the microscope, advances were also made in breast tumor characterization. The possible genetic basis of cancer was documented. The "seed and soil theory" was proposed by Stephen Paget. First attempts of reconstructive surgery for breast cancer were made. The bases of radiotherapy, immunotherapy and endocrine therapy were thrown.

During the 19th century, theory of cancer was revolutionized. Two German pathologists, Johannes Müller (1801-1858) and his student Rudolph *Ludwig Carl* Virchow (1821-1902), triggered the revolution.

Müller demonstrated that cancer is made up of cells and not lymph. However, he was of the opinion that cancer cells did not arise from normal cells, but from budding elements, called *blastema*, scattered between normal tissue components. German physician Hermann Lebert (1813-1878), a strong believer in this *blastema* theory, went as far as claiming with others, that there is no need to have an organ to produce cancer. The only thing needed is a capillary vessel with blood in it (in [Hajdu 2006]).

Rudolph Virchow, the dominant figure in German medical research for half a century, disproved the *blastema* theory by demonstrating that cancer cells are derived from other cells ("Omnis Cellula e Cellula" - every cell arises from another cell-). However, Virchow falsely held the view that metastatic cancers are spread by a liquid and that axillary metastases arose from cells in the nodes responding to "hurtful ingredients" or "poisonous matter" produced by the primary lesion.

German surgeon Karl (or Carl) Thiersch (1822-1895) went on to show that metastatic cancers arise not from a liquid but from the spread of malignant cells. In 1865, Thiersch proved that skin cancer begins as a primary focus, and that metastases result from lymphatic and vascular dissemination. In 1872, German anatomist *Heinrich* Wilhelm *Gottfriedvon* Waldeyer-*Hartz* (1836-1921) confirmed that it was true for all types of cancer, including breast cancer. Consequently, in the 19th century, the lymph and *blastema* theories were disproved and replaced by the modern cellular theory of cancer. One important consequence is that surgeons began to use frozen biopsy sections for examination under the microscope during surgery.

Virchow was convinced that carcinomas derive from immature cells scattered through the connective tissue, but soon was disproved by the studies of Victor *André* Cornil (1837-1908), Thiersch, and Waldeyer (1836-1921). Still, no clue was provided to explain the invasion of the epithelium. Julius *Friedriech* Cohnheim (1839-1884) and Hugo Ribbert (1855-1920) hypothesized that invasion of epithelia was only possible in the case of a primarily altered connective tissue. Ultimately the stroma determines malignant growth. From 1902, Max Borst (1869-1946) finally formulated the views on tumor-stroma-relationship which are still valid today. He also postulated interrelationships between tumor and stroma, which nowadays can be proven using molecular biological approaches [Dhom 1994].

Virchow studied aspects of inflammation and went to the conclusion that chronic inflammation is a pre-disposing factor for tumor genesis. Virchow noted the association between inflammation and cancer and suggested that the two processes were related (the "irritation hypothesis").

In contrast to Galen, Virchow did not regard breast cancer as systemic at onset, but rather a local disease, amenable to cure with surgery. Virchow's theory had a profound influence on the American surgeon William *Stewart* Halsted (1852-1922), who travelled through Europe in the late 19th century and studied with many of Virchow's pupils. If Virchow may be regarded as the architect of the new cellular theory on breast cancer pathogenesis, then Halsted should be viewed as its engineer.

Italian statistician Domenico *Antonio* Rigoni-Stern (1810-1855), had the morbid duty of perusing death certificates.Using analyses by age, sex and occupation, he noticed an odd discrepancy in cancer rates for women of various social positions [Rigoni-Stern 1842]. He observed that the higher frequency of breast cancer was between the 6th and 7th decades, that breast cancer was five times more frequent in nuns than among other women and that it was more common in the left than in the right breast. Rigoni-Stern speculated that the high incidence of breast cancer among members of religious orders might be due to excessive use of fish or garlic, or long periods of abstinence; or possibly to the effects of pressure from corsets or prolonged kneeling.

The results of surgery for breast cancer in the mid-19th century were still poor, partly because virtually all breast cancers diagnosed were locally advanced and there was a high operative mortality (up to 20%) due to overwhelming infection. The aggressive surgical treatment of breast cancer was considered unwise by many due in no small part to the lack of asepsis and anesthesia. Even those patients who survived rarely lived longer than 2 years. English surgeon James Paget (1814-1899) confessed to never having seen a cure of breast cancer.

Crawford *Williamson* Long (1815-1878) was the first to use ether as an anesthesic, in 1842. However, although Long demonstrated its use to physicians in Georgia on numerous occasions, he did not publish his findings until 1849, in The Southern Medical and Surgical Journal. The first to publicly demonstrate, in 1846, the use of ether as an anesthesic during an operation was the dentist William *Thomas Green* Morton (1819-1868). This set the stage for more ambitious surgical techniques. After the introduction of anesthesia in the 1840s, Joseph Lister (1827–1912) developed the concept of antisepsis using carbolic acid. Lister's rationale was based on Louis Pasteur's (1822-1895) theory that bacteria caused infection. He countered post-operative wound infections such as tetanus, blood-poisoning, and gangrene by using lint soaked in carbolic acid around the wound and replaced silk stitching with cat-gut ligatures which absorbed the carbolic acid more easily. Anesthesia and antisepsis (later asepsis) allowed surgery to be done more safely on an elective basis. Another important advance in surgery was the introduction of rubber gloves. Caroline Hampton (1861-1922), William Halsted's operating-room nurse and wife-to-be, developed dermatitis from the disinfectants in the operating room. Halsted asked the Goodyear Rubber Company to make special thin gloves for her. Gloves were introduced in 1889 and soon the entire operating room staff at John Hopkins Hospital was wearing them. They were to play an important role in surgical asepsis.

French surgeon and anatomist Alfred *Louis Armand Marie* Velpeau (1795-1867) was not only the inventor of the well-known "Velpeau's bandage", a bandage which serves to immobilize arm to chest wall, with the forearm positioned obliquely across and upward on front of chest. He was also the first to describe breast cancer "en cuirasse", the deadly form that spreads across the chest like a breast plate. His "Traité Des Maladies Du Sein Et De La Région Mammaire" ("A Treatise on the Diseases of the Breast and Mammary Region"), published in 1854, was a comprehensive review of breast disease of the time.

The possible genetic basis of cancer was first documented by Brazilian ophthalmologist Hilário *Soares* de Gouvêa (1843-1923), who reported about a family with retinoblastoma in more than one generation. Regarding breast cancer, its possible hereditary nature, suspected for centuries, was first described in details in 1866 by the French surgeon Pierre Paul Broca (1824-1880). He described an excess of breast cancer in multiple generations of his wife's family.

Advances in the development of the microscope have kick-started the science of cancer. In 1871, the first clinical paper written by Canadian physician William Osler (1849-1919), while still a medical student, described the gross, but also the microscopic findings of a patient with breast cancer (in [Stone 2003]).

Before the introduction of cellular theory of cancer, surgeons were often reluctant to operate, because it was felt from the beginning that cancer was a generalized and multicentric disease. Based on the works of Thiersch and Waldeyer, it became clear that cancer began as a local disease, with subsequent metastatic complications which should be avoided as early as possible. The way to radical mastectomy was opened.

As early as 1844, American surgeon Joseph Pancoast (1805-1882) recommended removal of the breast and glands all in one piece. In 1867, Charles Hewitt Moore (1821-1870) published a paper in which he observed that recurrences after limited operations for breast cancer were generally near the scar and that their pattern suggested centrifugal spread from the original site [Moore, 1867]. His principles of surgical cure were to remove the whole breast (including as much skin as was felt to be 'unsound'), avoiding cutting into the tumor, and removal of diseased axillary glands as advocated by Peyrihle nearly 100 years earlier. In fact, Moore initially recommended excising only clinically enlarged axillary but then realized the difficulty in knowing whether the glands were involved or not and stated that they can never be assumed to be normal. The anterior wall of the axilla is composed of the pectoralis major and minor muscle and the fascia that covers them. Moore recommended removal of pectoral muscles if they were involved. Indeed, with the advent of the microscope and developments in pathological anatomy, it was that the pectoralis fascia was occasionally microscopically involved with tumor not obvious to the naked eye.

Moore's procedure rapidly became the standard operation in Germany and Austria, after Richard von Volkmann (1830-1889) introduced a similar operation in 1873. In Volkmann's clinic, between 1874 and 1878, 11% of 200 patients treated were alive 3 years later. Samuel *Weissel* Gross (1837-1889) introduced Moore's principles in the USA, performing axillary dissections in every case. Routine axillary excision and dissection was also advocated by German Ernst *Georg Ferdinand* Küster (1839–1930) and Scottish William *Mitchell* Banks (1842-1904) [Banks 1882]. The removal of the entire pectoralis muscle if the cancer was infiltrating part of the fascia or muscle was advocated by Lothar Heidenhain (1860-1940) [Heidenhain 1889].

All of this served as a prelude, when, in 1882, William Stewart Halsted (1852-1922), applying the philosophy and techniques of Moore and his disciples, began to perform the first radical mastectomy, or the en bloc removal of the entire breast, regional lymphatics, and entire pectoralis major. At once, Halsted obtained results that far exceeded any that had been obtained by his predecessors. On the first series of 50 patients, a dramatic fall in local recurrence to 6% compared with the 56–81% reported in Europe was observed [Halsted 1894]. When Halsted presented his series of 133 patients to the American Surgical Association, in 1898, the 3-year survival rate was 53%, with a local recurrence of 9%. The radical mastectomy was an operation whose time had arrived [Cotlar *et al.* 2003] and Halsted's impressive results would totally revolutionize the surgical approach to breast cancer, and influence treatment for three-quarters of a century.

The correlation of the clinical behavior of a tumor with its histologic type and treatment outcome was illustrated in the 1870's, notably by German-Austrian surgeon *Christian Albert* Theodor Billroth (1829-1894) and his Austrian-Belgian assistant Alexander von Winiwarter (1848-1917). They analyzed an enormous amount of raw statistical data related to breast cancer. This enabled them to correlate age with certain types of breast cancer and to also predict its outcome. From these data they postulated that medullary carcinoma had the most rapid course and was more likely to occur in younger women. Carcinoma simplex was the most frequent, but had an unpredictable clinical course. Aggressive neoplasms were more frequent in young women between 30 and 40 in otherwise good health. Von Winiwarter published a study in 1878, based on data obtained from Billroth's follow up of breast cancer surgery, which was used to justify surgical intervention with the aim of cure. It demonstrated that 4.7% of 170 cancer patients who had their tumors excised were in fact alive after three years.

The end of 19th century was characterized by first attempts of reconstructive surgery for breast cancer. In 1895, Vinzenz Czerny (1842-1916) transplanted a large fatty tumor (a lipoma), removed from the lumbar region of the patient, to replace a breast that has been surgically removed. One year later, Iginio Tansini (1855-1943) reported the first radical mastectomy with reconstructive surgery using a flap made from muscle and skin.

In 1877, Russian veterinarian Mstislav *Aleksandrovich* Novinsky (1841-1914) successfully transplanted 2 tumors, a nasal tumor and a venereal myxosarcoma, in dogs, but this was reported in an incomplete, preliminary paper [Shimkin 1960]. In 1889, the German pathologist Arthur *Nathan* Hanau (1858-1900) realized the homologous transplantation of a rat vulvar epidermoid carcinoma. Modern experimental oncology was born.

It had been observed in the 19th century that the growth of breast cancer in patients sometimes fluctuated with the menstrual cycle and that the disease grew more slowly in postmenopausal women. In 1882, Thomas *William* Nunn (1825-1909) described a case of breast cancer remission occurring 6 months after menopause. In 1889, German surgeon Albert Schinzinger (1827-1911) first proposed surgical oophorectomy as a treatment for breast cancer patients, but did not perform it [Schinzinger 1889]. In 1878, *George* Thomas Beatson (1848-1933) had discovered that the breasts of rabbits stopped producing milk after he removed the ovaries, indicating that some aspects of breast activity were under ovarian control. In 1896, he described temporary regression of metastatic breast cancer in two patients treated by surgical oophorectomy [Beatson 1896]. Thus, Beatson had discovered the stimulating effect of estrogens long before the hormone was identified. Beatson's work is the basis for today's hormone therapy, as well as the development of such drugs as tamoxifen.

Stephen Paget (1855-1926), in his "seed and soil" theory (1889), proposed that cancer cells ("seed") travel through the body via the bloodstream where they are able to grow in certain "compatible" organs ("soil"). This theory of metastasis foresaw the limitations of surgery for curing advanced (metastatic) breast cancer.

In the 1890s, William *Bradley* Coley (1862-1936) reported on injections of bacterial extracts from organisms causing erysipelas (streptococci) that resulted in regression of advanced cancers. These extracts, known as "Coley's toxins," generated much controversy (reviewed in [Wiemann and Starnes 1994]). While Coley's toxins were shown to produce high responses rates in sarcoma, the responses were generally not as good in other types of cancer, usually carcinomas [Tsung and Norton 2006]. Coley's work is now seen as one of the earliest attempts at immunotherapy of cancer by stimulating the host's immune system. Nearly a century later, interest in this type of approach was revived with the discovery of tumor necrosis factor and other immune-stimulating cytokines. It has been recently suggested that the active molecule in Coley's toxin is interleukin-12 [Tsung and Norton 2006].

The last major revolution brought by the 19th century was initiated by Wilhelm *Conrad* Röntgen (1845-1923) and the Curie, Pierre (1859-1906) and Marie (1867-1934). In 1895, Röntgen accidentally discovered X-rays. In the same year, the French Victor Despeignes (1866-1937) announced the first X-rays treatment to a patient in France. In 1898 the Curie discovered the radioactive element radium. In 1899, Tage *Anton Ultimus* Sjogren (1859-1939) became the first person to successfully treat cancer with X-rays. In 1900,Thor *Johan* Stenbeck (1864-1914) cured a patient with skin cancer using small doses of daily radiation therapy. This technique was later referred to as fractionated radiation therapy.

References

Banks WM. On Free Removal of Mammary Cancer, with Extirpation of the Axillary Glands as a Necessary Accompaniment. *Br. Med. J.* 1882 December 9;2(1145):1138–41.

Beatson GT. On the treatment of inoperable cases of carcinoma of the mamma: suggestions for a new method of treatment, with illustrative cases. *Lancet* 1896;2:104–7 and 162-5.

Cotlar AM, Dubose JJ, Rose DM. History of surgery for breast cancer: radical to the sublime. *Curr. Surg.* 2003 May-Jun;60(3):329-37.

Dhom G. [The cancer cell and the connective tissue. A historical retrospect] (german) *Pathologe.* 1994 Oct;15(5):271-8.

Hajdu SI. Thoughts about the cause of cancer. *Cancer.* 2006 Apr 15;106(8):1643-9.

Halsted WS. I. The Results of Operations for the Cure of Cancer of the Breast Performed at the Johns Hopkins Hospital from June, 1889, to January, 1894. *Ann. Surg.* 1894 Nov;20(5):497-555.

Heidenhain L.Ueber die ursachen der localen krebsrecidive nach amputatio mammae. *Arch. Klin. Chir.* 1889;39:97–166.

Moore CH. On the influence of inadequate operations on the theory of cancer. *Roy. Med. Chir. Soc. Lond.* 1867;1:244–80.

Rigoni-Stern D. Fatti statistici relativi alle malattie cancerose che servirono de base alle poche cose dette dal dott. *Gior. Servire. Progr. Pat. Terap.* 1842;2:507-17.

Schinzinger A. Ueber carcinoma mammae [abstract]. 18th Congress of the German Society for Surgery. Beilage zum Zentralblatt fur Chirurgie. 1889;16: 55-6

Shimkin MB. Arthur Nathan Hanau: a further note on the history of transplantation of tumors. *Cancer.* 1960 Mar-Apr;13:221.

Stone MJ. William Osler's legacy and his contribution to haematology. *Br. J. Haematol.* 2003 Oct;123(1):3-18.

Tsung K, Norton JA. Lessons from Coley's Toxin. *Surg. Oncol.* 2006 Jul;15(1):25-8.

Wiemann B, Starnes CO. Coley's toxins, tumor necrosis factor and cancer research: a historical perspective. *Pharmacol. Ther.* 1994;64(3):529-64.

Chapter 4

Twentieth Century and Beyond Breast Cancer Surgery

Abstract

In the first half of the 20th century, surgery was dominated by the principles of William Halsted and supported by the view that cancer was a local-regional disease spreading in an orderly fashion based on mechanical considerations. Halsted's followers continued to espouse his principles and performed even more extensive mastectomies. However, starting in the 1960's, this approach was progressively challenged, based on laboratory and clinical research supporting the idea that operable cancer was a systemic disease. Simple mastectomy was reintroduced. Currently, breast-conserving surgery is performed in most cases. Other advances in surgery include mammary reconstruction, minimally invasive surgery and the use of sentinel lymph node.

In the 19th century, as mentioned in chapter 3, the humoral and lymph theories of cancer were progressively supplanted by the cellular theory, mainly as a consequence of Virchow's work. According to the view that breast cancer may appear locally, before disseminating in the body, increasingly aggressive surgical approaches were developed in the end of the 19th century and during the first half of the 20th century [Jatoi 1997].

In Halsted's radical mastectomy, the tumor-containing breast, underlying muscles (entire pectoralis major), and ipsilateral axillary contents were removed *en bloc*. In this manner, the lymphatic channels connecting the breast and axillary contents were extirpated, a clear acceptance of the teachings of Virchow and a repudiation of the systemic hypothesis concerning breast cancer pathogenesis.

Halsted's operation was supported conceptually by the centrifugal permeation theory proposed by English surgeon William Sampson Handley (1872–1962). This theory stated that cancers originated at one focus and spread from it exclusively through lymphatics. This lymphatic spread was by growth in continuity (permeation) rather than embolic spread and occurred equally in all directions. Regional lymph nodes halted the progress of permeation only temporarily, but thereafter growth through the lymph nodes allowed haematogenous embolization and dissemination in the body.

In 1894, Willie Meyer (1858–1932), reported a slightly different operation [Meyer 1894]. The differences in details of the operative technique were that Meyer used a diagonal incision, dissected the axillary contents first and excised pectoralis minor, a modification which Halsted subsequently adopted. Meyer left enough skin to ensure that the flaps could always be closed, whereas Halsted routinely used a skin graft to cover the defect. Another prominent surgeon, William *Louis* Rodman (1858-1916), supported Meyer's technique, including axillary dissection first, to minimize dissemination of tumor cells [Cotlar *et al.* 2003].In the beginning of 20th century, many surgeons had accepted the radical mastectomy. It is no doubt that the great effectiveness of this operation in achieving local control of this disease contributed to its immense popularity.

The main achievement of Halsted's operation was the reduction of local recurrence rates compared with lesser operations, but it became clear subsequently that little had been achieved in terms of overall survival. This may in part have been due to the fact that many patients who underwent radical mastectomy had relatively advanced disease. The contraindications to radical mastectomy were subsequently defined by Cushman *Davis* Haagensen (1900-1990) with improved results in terms of local recurrence and overall survival in line with better case selection and earlier diagnosis. Haagensen is known to have originated the Columbia Clinical Classification (CCC) staging system (see chapter 9).

In 1927, William Sampson Handley reported that internal mammary lymph nodes often contain breast cancer metastases [Handley 1927]. Twenty-two years later, in 1949, his son, Richard Sampson Handley (1909-1984), and pathologist Alan *Christopher* Thackray (1914-2004) described 50 consecutive patients who underwent mastectomy plus removal of ipsilateral internal mammary lymph nodes through the second intercostal space; 38% of them had internal mammary lymph node metastases [Handley and Thackray 1949]. Such observations of frequent lymph node involvement in breast cancer patients contributed to the extension of Halsted's operation, although it must be noted that William Sampson Handley suggested placement of radium tubes in the intercostal spaces rather than extended mastectomy (see chapter 5: radiotherapy).

However, until the 1960s, radiation therapy was not widely used in Western countries, and effective chemotherapy was not yet available. The most useful cancer-fighting tool was the scalpel.

Beginning in the late 1940's, there was a trend to more and more drastic surgery, fuelled by technological advances, such as improvements in anesthetics and blood transfusion and the use of antibiotics. The radical mastectomy was extended by a number of surgeons to include removal of internal mammary lymph nodes, as exemplified by Mario Margottini (1897-1971) [Margottini 1952; Margottini 1959], Umberto Veronesi (b. 1925) and Pietro Bucalossi (1905-1992) [Bucalossi and Veronesi 1959] in Italy, Eduardo Cáceres Graziani (b. 1915) [Cáceres 1959] in Peru, Everett *Dornbush* Sugarbaker (1910-2001) and Jerome *Andrew* Urban (1914-1991) [Sugarbaker 1953; Urban 1964] in the USA.

This "extended radical mastectomy" was extended even further to include removal of the supraclavicular lymph nodes at the time of mastectomy. This was notably performed by Erling Dahl-Iversen (1892-1978) in Denmark [Andreassen *et al.* 1954; Dahl-Iversen and Tobiassen 1969]. Owen *Harding* Wangensteen (1898-1981) in Minnesota added removal of mediastinal nodes ("super-radical mastectomy") [Wangensteen 1957]. Other than showing that extra-axillary nodes often contained metastases and that their removal improved regional tumor control, cures were not increased.

Indeed, randomized, controlled studies have found no difference in overall survival between the radical mastectomy and extended or super-radical mastectomy [Veronesi and Valagussa1981; Lacour *et al.* 1983; Lacour *et al.* 1987], and these extensions, often accompanied by a significant operative mortality, were eventually abandoned in favor of chest wall and regional irradiation.

Prophylactic simple mastectomy was also proposed for the other breast (contralateral) at the time of radical mastectomy. This operation was first advocated in 1921 by Joseph *Colt* Bloodgood (1867–1935), to reduce the risk for a second primary breast cancer [Bloodgood 1921].

Currently, prophylactic mastectomy (PM) is an option for BRCA1/BRCA2 carriers (see chapter 10) and other high-risk women: in such cases, bilateral PM may be performed on women who have not had cancer, while contralateral PM is performed in women who had a therapeutic mastectomy for a primary cancer.

During the Halsted era, surgeons generally assumed that the radical mastectomy reduced breast cancer mortality. This assumption was based on the observation that the radical mastectomy was very effective in achieving local control of the disease, and it was believed that local control influenced survival. By the latter half of the twentieth century, this assumption was increasingly questioned.

Of note, starting from the early 1920's, less debilitating operations accompanied by radiotherapy had been advocated by William Handley, Roy Ward, Geoffrey Keynes, and Robert McWhirter, among others. For more details, see chapter 5).

In 1948, David *Howard* Patey (1899-1977) described a modification of the Halsted mastectomy [Patey and Dyson 1948]. In this "modified radical mastectomy," the pectoralis major muscle was preserved. The operation was less debilitating, and the authors reported that its results were as good as those of the standard radical procedure.

Many surgeons, such as John *Leo* Madden (1912-1999) [Madden 1965] and Hugh Auchincloss (1915-1998) [Auchincloss 1970] in the USA, and Richard Handley in Europe soon adopted this procedure as an alternative to the more radical Halsted operation. By 1981, modified radical mastectomy was performed in 77.1% of cases of diagnosed breast cancer, and the use of radical mastectomy had decreased to 3.4%. Indeed, the modified radical mastectomy (with preservation of both the pectoralis major and minor muscles) is still widely used today in the treatment of early breast cancer.

In 1951, Canadian physician Ian MacDonald produced data indicating that prompt treatment was much less important than the biology of the individual breast cancer ("biological predeterminism") [MacDonald 1951]. Thus, even some small tumors could be fatal due to their rapid dissemination. These data challenged Halsted's belief that early, aggressive intervention cures more cancers and concluded there was often little that the medical profession could do to alter the fate of cancer patients.

MacDonald claimed many surgeons are carrying out pointless surgical treatments for cancers that are already destined to be lethal.

Still in 1951, two biometricians, Scottish *William* Wallace Park (1916-1998) and English James Lees, after reviewing the published literature on breast cancer, estimated that radical mastectomy actually improved survival from breast cancer in only 5 to 10 percent of cases [Park and Lees 1951].

In 1953, English surgeon Reginald Murley (1916-1997) and radiotherapist Ivor *Glyn* Williams (1913-1995) analyzed case records of patients treated twenty to thirty years earlier by Geoffrey Keynes (see chapter 5). They were surprised to find that patients treated with simple excision and radiation therapy survive as long as those treated at the same hospital by radical surgery.

In 1955, young American surgeon George Crile Jr (1907-1992), a supporter of radical surgery, was persuaded by Murley's data analyses and abruptly stopped performing the technique in favor of breast-conserving surgery (simple mastectomy or, in early stages, lumpectomy, in which the tumor and a minimal amount of surrounding tissue is removed by a local incision) [Crile 1972].

He was seen as an "extremist" and attacked by most colleagues (see for instance the editorial of Warfield *Monroe* Firor (1896-1988) in 1960 [Firor 1960] and the response of Crile [Crile 1960]). George Crile criticized the approach to educating the public through fear. His decision to publish an article aimed at the general public (women's magazine) on this was condemned by the medical profession.

Besides George Crile, another American surgeon, Oliver Cope (1902-1994) abandoned radical surgical treatments of breast cancer [Cope *et al.* 1972], went outside of the medical community and began to write for the popular media in the early 1970's, in order to reach a wider audience.

In the second half of the 20th century, it was clear that radical surgery was unable to cure breast cancer in over a third of patients.

A greater awareness of postoperative morbidity such as deformity of the chest, lymphedema of the arm and occasional irradiation-induced sarcomas led to some surgeons becoming increasingly critical of radical surgery and led to a reevaluation of less radical surgery for breast cancer.

This also reflected the fact that an increasing percentage of women diagnosed with breast cancer also objected to radical operations and at times insisted upon lesser procedures.

Another objection to radical surgery resulted from the enormous explosion of knowledge about the biology of breast cancer, killing off old theories of cancer spread and redefining the indications for surgery.

"Halstedian hypothesis" was replaced by the "biological hypothesis", also named "Fisher hypothesis", since physician Bernard Fisher (b. 1918) was a major contributor [Fisher 2008]. The comparison between Halstedian and biological hypotheses is summarized in Table 1.

Table 1. Comparison of Halstedian and biological hypotheses of tumor progression. The biological theory now is basis for all our treatment concepts, where adjuvant (postoperative) or neoadjuvant (preoperative) systemic treatment (see chapter 6) is standard of care

Halstedian hypothesis	Biological hypothesis
Tumors spread in an orderly defined manner based upon mechanical considerations	There is no orderly pattern of tumor cell dissemination
Tumor cells traverse lymphatics to lymph nodes by direct extension	Tumor cells traverse lymphatics by embolization
The positive lymph node is an indicator of tumor spread and is the instigator of distant disease	The positive lymph node is an indicator of a host–tumor relationship which permits development of metastases rather than the instigator of distant disease
Regional lymph nodes are barriers to the passage of tumor cells	Regional lymph nodes are ineffective as barriers to tumor cell spread
Regional lymph nodes are of anatomical importance	Regional lymph nodes are of biological importance
The blood stream is of little significance as a route of tumor dissemination	The blood stream is of considerable importance in tumor dissemination
A tumor is autonomous of its host	Complex tumor–host interrelationships affect every facet of the disease.
Operable breast cancer is a local–regional disease	Operable breast cancer is a systemic disease
The extent and nuances of operation are the dominant factors influencing patient outcome	Variations in local–regional therapy are unlikely to substantially affect survival

Starting in the 1960's, a vast series of randomized and controlled trials of breast-sparing surgery compared to radical surgery or simple mastectomy were performed. The first of such studies began in 1961 at Guy's Hospital (London). The study compared tumor wide local removal in conjunction with low-dose radiotherapy against radical mastectomy. It initially found equivalent 10-year survival rates in the two procedures for patients with stage I disease. Unfortunately, cancer cells had spread to the axillary lymph nodes in many stage II patients, resulting in extensive local recurrences and significantly worse survival in the tumor local excision and radiotherapy group (reported in [Atkins *et al.* 1972]). The results were widely publicized and the conservative surgery movement was set back.

However, in the following decades, a series of retrospective studies and of prospective randomized clinical trials ([Veronesi *et al.* 1981; Fisher *et al.*1985, Fisher *et al.* 1989, Sarrazin *et al.* 1989; Straus *et al.* 1992, Blichert-Toft *et al.* 1992, Lichter *et al.* 1992, Fisher *et al.* 1995; Jacobson *et al.* 1995, Arriagada *et al.* 1996, van Dongen *et al.* 2000, Veronesi *et al.* 2002, Fisher *et al.* 2002]) indicated that breast-conserving surgery and mastectomy produce similar results in terms of regional control and survival. These studies have established breast-conserving therapy as the preferred treatment of early stages (stages I and II) breast cancer (see notably [National Institutes of Health Consensus Development Panel Consensus Statement 1992]).

However, not all patients with early breast cancer are suitable for breast-conserving techniques (see below), and other factors which need to be taken into account when considering the type of surgery as the initial treatment are the size of the tumor in relation with the size of the breast and the location of the tumor in relation to the nipple-areolar complex.

In parallel, the changes in breast cancer hypothesis led the scientists to develop medications that would kill the malignant cells that had spread through the body. This was the beginning of chemotherapeutic approaches (see chapter 6).

Finally, increased patient awareness and education, the introduction of mass screening, and advances in high-quality mammography, resulted in earlier diagnosis of breast cancer and the detection of asymptomatic lesions.

Although the diagnosis of breast cancer was more frequently made, the size of the primary lesion and extent of axillary node metastasis, diminished [Cotlar *et al.* 2003], supporting the use of breast-conserving therapy.

After 1980, breast conservation, supported by good-quality, prospective, randomized controlled trials, became much more widely utilized as combined modality therapy.

Currently, nearly all women with small invasive breast cancers can opt for breast conservation surgery and can be treated as an outpatient. This experience is in clear contrast with that of a woman undergoing extended radical mastectomy (with removal of the breast, chest muscles and ribs, see above).

Recent Evolutions in Breast Cancer Surgery

A) Mammary Reconstruction

During the last 50 years, plastic surgeons have taken a special interest in mammary reconstruction.

In 1942, New Zealander Harold *Delf* Gillies (1882-1960) used tubed pedicle technique for breast reconstruction.

In 1963, two plastic surgeons, AmericanThomas *Dillon* Cronin (1906-1993) and Canadian Frank *Judson* Gerow (1929-1993) used silicone for breast reconstruction, with more satisfying results than previous methods.

In the 1970s, the crucial work of German Carl Manchot (1866-1932) on vascular territories led to the use of flaps in breast reconstruction. The earliest techniques to allow for breast reconstruction using natural tissues from a woman's body rather than an artificial implant utilized muscles to provide blood flow to skin and fat so that that this tissue could be transported to the chest to create a breast mound. The *latissimus dorsi* flap was the most popular form of autogenous tissue breast cancer reconstruction in the 1970s. Skin, fat and muscle from the back were rotated to the front of the body to create a breast. Today, this procedure is used in conjunction with implants to provide a fuller looking breast.

In 1982, the first *transverse rectus abdominus myocutaneous* (TRAM) flap reconstruction was performed. In this procedure, a woman's lower abdominal skin and fat is used to make the breast. In this flap, the *rectus abdominis* muscle is used to support the skin and fat which is tunneled up into the breast area. Today, this flap remains the standard of care, creating natural appearing breasts and improved abdominal contours.

Nevertheless, there are drawbacks to using these muscles and so techniques have evolved to minimize or eliminate the need for sacrificing muscles for breast cancer reconstruction. The use of microvascular free flaps allows transplanting tissue from one part of the body to another without the use of a large muscle.

The abdomen is the source of many varieties of such flaps. The TRAM free flap uses only a small portion of the rectus muscle, while the *deep inferior epigastric perforator* (DIEP) free flap, and the *superficial inferior epigastric artery* (SIEA) free flap utilize none of the rectus muscle.

The buttock is another source of skin and fat that can be used to create a breast. The *gluteal artery perforator* (GAP) free flaps allow a hidden donor site most useful for women with insufficient abdominal tissue. As a result of these procedures, women recover easier and have fewer complications from the donor site.

In 1988, the FDA classified breast implants as a high-risk product and demanded that manufacturers prove that they are safe and effective to use. A gradual shift from silicone to saline implants begins taking place in the US and Canada.

Finally, in November of 2006, the FDA reversed its ban on silicone-filled breast implants. Now, silicone gel implants are widely used for both cosmetic breast augmentation and breast cancer reconstruction. Both saline and silicone implants are popular choices today.

B) Sentinel Lymph Node Mapping

The concept of sentinel lymph node (SLN) was initially developed by Ramón *Maximino* Cabanas, studying penile cancer [Cabanas 1977].

In breast cancer, axillary SLN biopsy was introduced in the 1990's, as a means improving quality of life in patients with primary breast cancer.SLN is the first lymph node (LN) in the axillary basin to receive metastases from the primary breast cancer if they have occurred [Giuliano *et al.* 1994]. By injecting a radioactive dye near the breast tumor, surgeons can pinpoint to which lymph node it drains. If the true SLN is negative, the chance of tumor in the remaining axillary LNs is less than 1%.

Therefore, it may be unnecessary to perform further axillary LN dissection (ALND), which is a cause of significant morbidity in terms of lymphedema, numbness to the arm, and decreased range of motion.

The assessment of the SLN at the time of initial diagnosis may improve upon the current staging molecular methods -multiple mRNA marker RT-PCR analysis, which would identify the sub-group of patients with metastases in the SLN but thought to be free of disease by conventional pathologic examinations [Kuerer and Newman 2005]. Large trials are currently underway comparing the efficacy of sentinel node biopsy to the standard ALND.

First studies, such as ALMANAC (Axillary Lymphatic Mapping Against Nodal Axillary Clearance), have suggested that SLN biopsy is associated with reduced arm morbidity and better quality of life than standard axillary treatment and should be the treatment of choice for patients who have early-stage breast cancer with clinically negative LNs [Mansel *et al.* 2006].

C) Biopsies: Evolution of Tissue Sampling Techniques

Since the 1960's, needle localization followed by open surgical biopsy has been usedas diagnostic procedure for suspected breast lesions. This involves marking of the lesion by a hooked wire under mammographic or ultrasound guidance, followed by wide surgical excision of the tissue surrounding the tip of the wire. After radiography confirms the presence of the lesion in the excised specimen, a final pathologic diagnosis can be established. This procedure is extremely accurate [Verkooijen *et al.* 2000], but associated morbidity and costs are high.

Mass screening has resulted in large numbers of nonpalpable lesions being suspected.The fact that up to 80%–90% of women with nonpalpable breast lesions turn out to have benign disease and, in retrospect, undergo unnecessary surgery, fuelled the development of minimally invasive procedures. Various percutaneous biopsy technique have been introduced: 1) fine needle aspiration, 2) large-core biopsy, and 3) vacuum-assisted breast biopsy; they are generally used with image guidance (ultrasound, stereotaxis or MRI).

1) Fine needle aspiration (FNA) has been used for the diagnosis of breast cancer since the mid-1970's. It is a well-established tool for the evaluation of palpable breast lumps (i.e. triple test involving clinical examination, imaging, and FNA) but is less suitable for diagnosis of nonpalpable breast cancer. FNA allows the pathologist to identify the presence of malignant cells but not to distinguish between invasive and in situ cancer. In addition, FNA suffers from high inadequate sampling and false-negative rates [Wells 1995].

2) The limitations of FNA led, in the early 1990's to the introduction of large-core needle biopsy for the diagnostic workup of nonpalpable breast lesions. With large-core needle biopsy, actual tissue samples are obtained by means of a large-core needle (generally 14-gauge) and an automated biopsy gun. A minimum of four samples is needed, and for lesions containing microcalcifications, specimen radiography is essential in verifying the adequacy of sampling. Large-core needle biopsy is less operator-dependent than FNA. Because it obtains an actual tissue sample, it allows identification of an invasive

component. It facilitates the assessment of tumor grade and provides sufficient material for additional immunochemistry staining. Diagnostic accuracy of large-core needle biopsy is high. However, in some cases, the severity of the disease is underestimated (see references in [Vlastos and Verkooijen 2007])..

3) In an attempt to reduce disease underestimate rates, vacuum-assisted breast biopsy was introduced in 1995. With this technique, tissue samples are acquired by using a single insertion of a probe (generally 11-gauge) and vacuum suction to retrieve core specimens. Advantages are that more material can be obtained in a shorter period of time and that only one single insertion of the biopsy probe is needed. However, the costs of vacuum-assisted breast biopsy are substantially higher than those of large core needle biopsy, so that it may not be cost-effective for routine use (see references in [Vlastos and Verkooijen 2007]).

D) Minimally Invasive Surgery

It is increasingly suggested that minimally invasive surgery approaches used for biopsies could also be used for the treatment of early-stage cancers and benign tumors of the breast. Five different procedures are currently studied: percutaneous stereotactic excision, radiofrequency ablation, focused ultrasound ablation, laser ablation, and cryotherapy. The last four techniques use either local freezing or heat to cause cell death and tumor destruction. These techniques are currently under development and appear to be safe, as only few complications such as infection, bleeding, or skin burns are described (see references in [Vlastos and Verkooijen 2007]).

1) Percutaneous stereotactic biopsy techniques have been used as a treatment option for excision of benign and malignant breast lesions [Fine *et al.* 2003]. Various stereotactic biopsy systems, based on different technologies (vacuum assisted core biopsy or large core biopsy), were developed and subsequently used in a percutaneous excisional purpose. The sensitivity and specificity of these systems for the diagnosis of breast cancer are both excellent. It has been shown that the positive margins and residual tumor rates are comparable to those obtained with the use of wire-localized excisional biopsies. However, an important disadvantage is the impossibility to evaluate

tumor margins. Prospective multicenter studies are needed to evaluate the efficacy and cost-effectiveness of these different percutaneous excision techniques (see references in [Vlastos and Verkooijen 2007]).

2) Radiofrequency ablation (RFA) destroys early-stage tumors with heat. Under imaging (generally ultrasound) guidance, a radiofrequency probe (15-gauge) with a star-like array of RFA electrodes is inserted in the tumor, and an alternating high-frequency electric current (400–500 kHz) is administered. The heat that is generated at 95°C leads to the interruption of cell replication and triggered irreversible tumor destruction, as tumor cells are more susceptible to heat than are normal cells. Fifteen minutes are needed to achieve complete ablation, which is signaled by a coagulated opaque area (hyperechoic) of about 2 cm can be visualized with ultrasound. In the surgical specimen, this area macroscopically appears as a yellow-white appearance and is surrounded by a red rim. Since 1999, several studies evaluated the use of RFA ablation in the treatment of breast cancer. They concluded that breast tumors were ablated in a high percentage of cases (see references in [Vlastos and Verkooijen 2007]).

3) Focused ultrasound ablation (FUS) is another thermal method. Ultrasound are focused on the tumor and rapidly generate a substantial increase in local temperatures of up to 90°C by converting acoustic energy into heat. FUS ablation heats the tumor and causes cell damage and tumor death. Tumor ablation is monitored through temperature probes and skin monitors. Ten minutes are usually needed to complete ablation. Very small lesions can be targeted by this approach. Therefore, high-resolution imaging techniques, such as MRI, need to be used for accurate detection and monitoring. The major advantage of FUS over other ablative techniques is that no skin incisions are needed. However, tumors close to the skin may be treated with less success and with such adverse effects as skin burns. Recent FUS studies on breast tumors have shown that it was effective, safe and feasible (see references in [Vlastos and Verkooijen 2007]).

4) Laser ablation is a technique that generates heat and subsequently causes cell death and tumor destruction. Laser energy is delivered directly to the target tumor through a fiberoptic probe inserted under imaging guidance. Laser ablation consists in delivering 2–2.5 W in 500 s on the tumor. Laser treatments may be performed under imaging guidance (mammography, ultrasound, or MRI). A target

temperature of 80°C–100°C is generated during 15–20 minutes to obtain tumor ablation. Laser ablation for the treatment of early-stage breast cancer has not been studied extensively, but some have shown that small tumors can be ablated with negative margins (see references in [Vlastos and Verkooijen 2007]).

5) Cryotherapy uses coldness to achieve tumor destruction. Energy is produced by an external generator composed of an argon or nitrogen freezing system and a helium heating system. Cryosurgery involves the use of a freezing probe inserted in the center of the tumor under imaging guidance (ultrasound or MRI) through a tiny incision. Once the probe is positioned correctly, an iceball is created at the needle tip. This iceball destroys the tumor as well as 5–10 mm of additional breast tissue surrounding the lesion. During each freeze cycle, temperatures from -185°C to +70°C are obtained and constantly monitored. The length and sequence of freeze cycles can be modulated depending on the tumor volume to be ablated. Tumor destruction can be monitored in real time under ultrasound or MRI. Successful breast cancer treatment by cryotherapy has been shown in several studies (see references in [Vlastos and Verkooijen 2007]). The technique is promising for small tumors (less than 10-15 mm) and seems more successful in treating invasive than in situ disease. Additional research is needed to overcome in situ residual disease.

References

Andreassen M, Dahl-Iversen E, Sørensen B. Glandular metastases in carcinoma of the breast; results of a more radical operation. *Lancet.* 1954 Jan 23;266(6804):176-8.

Arriagada R, Lê MG, Rochard F, Contesso G. Conservative treatment versus mastectomy in early breast cancer: patterns of failure with 15 years of follow-up data. Institut Gustave-Roussy Breast Cancer Group. *J. Clin. Oncol.* 1996 May;14(5):1558-64.

Atkins H, Hayward JL, Klugman DJ, Wayte AB. Treatment of early breast cancer: a report after ten years of a clinical trial. *Br. Med. J.* 1972 May 20;2(5811):423-9.

Auchincloss H. Modified radical mastectomy: why not? *Am. J. Surg.* 1970 May;119(5):506-9.

Blichert-Toft M, Rose C, Andersen JA, Overgaard M, Axelsson CK, Andersen KW, Mouridsen HT. Danish randomized trial comparing breast conservation therapy with mastectomy: six years of life-table analysis. Danish Breast Cancer Cooperative Group. *J. Natl. Cancer Inst. Monogr.* 1992;(11):19-25.

Bloodgood JC. The remaining breast after radical removal of the opposite side for carcinoma. Trans Southern Surg Assoc. 1921;34:223-41.

Bucalossi P, Veronesi U. Long-term results of radical mastectomy with removal of internal mammary chain. *Acta Unio Int. Contra. Cancrum.* 1959;15:1052-5.

Cabanas RM. An approach for the treatment of penile carcinoma.*Cancer.* 1977 Feb;39(2):456-66.

Caceres E. Radical mastectomy with resection of the internal mammary chain. *Acta Unio Int. Contra. Cancrum.* 1959;15:1061-7.

Cope O, Wang CA, Chu A, Wang CC, Schulz M, Castleman B, Long J, Sohier WD. Limited surgical excision as the basis of a comprehensive therapy for cancer of the breast. *Am. J. Surg.* 1976 Apr;131(4):400-7.

Cotlar AM, Dubose JJ, Rose DM. History of surgery for breast cancer: radical to the sublime. *Curr. Surg.* 2003 May-Jun;60(3):329-37.

Crile G Jr. A critique of Dr. Firor's editorial on breast cancer. *Am. Surg.* 1960 Oct;26:692-3.

Crile G Jr. Low incidence and morbidity of local recurrence after conservative operations for cancer of the breast. *Ann. Surg.* 1972 Feb;175(2):249-53.

Dahl-Iversen E, Tobiassen T. Radical mastectomy with parasternal and supraclavicular dissection for mammary carcinoma. *Ann. Surg.* 1969 Dec;170(6):889-91.

Fine RE, Whitworth PW, Kim JA, Harness JK, Boyd BA, Burak WE Jr. Low-risk palpable breast masses removed using a vacuum-assisted hand-held device. *Am. J. Surg.* 2003 Oct;186(4):362-7.

Firor WM. Regression in the treatment of mammary carcinoma. *Am. Surg.* 1960 Jan;26:63.

Fisher B, Redmond C, Fisher ER, Bauer M, Wolmark N, Wickerham DL, Deutsch M, Montague E, Margolese R, Foster R. Ten-year results of a randomized clinical trial comparing radical mastectomy and total mastectomy with or without radiation. *N. Engl. J. Med.* 1985 Mar 14;312(11):674-81.

Fisher B, Redmond C, Poisson R, Margolese R, Wolmark N, Wickerham L, Fisher E, Deutsch M, Caplan R, Pilch Y, et al. Eight-year results of a randomized clinical trial comparing total mastectomy and lumpectomy with or without irradiation in the treatment of breast cancer. *N. Engl. J. Med.* 1989 Mar 30;320(13):822-8.

Fisher B, Anderson S, Redmond CK, Wolmark N, Wickerham DL, Cronin WM. Reanalysis and results after 12 years of follow-up in a randomized clinical trial comparing total mastectomy with lumpectomy with or without irradiation in the treatment of breast cancer. *N. Engl. J. Med.* 1995 Nov 30;333(22):1456-61.

Fisher B, Anderson S, Bryant J, Margolese RG, Deutsch M, Fisher ER, Jeong JH, Wolmark N. Twenty-year follow-up of a randomized trial comparing total mastectomy, lumpectomy, and lumpectomy plus irradiation for the treatment of invasive breast cancer. *N. Engl. J. Med.* 2002 Oct 17;347(16):1233-41.

Fisher B. Biological research in the evolution of cancer surgery: a personal perspective. *Cancer Res.* 2008 Dec 15;68(24):10007-20.

Giuliano AE, Kirgan DM, Guenther JM, Morton DL. Lymphatic mapping and sentinel lymphadenectomy for breast cancer. *Ann. Surg.* 1994 Sep;220(3):391-8.

Handley WS. Parasternal invasion of the thorax in breast cancer and its suppression by the use of radium tubes as an operative precaution. *Surg.Gynec. and Obstet* 1927;45:721–8.

Handley RS, Thackray AC. The internal mammary lymph chain in carcinoma of the breast: study of 50 cases. *Lancet.* 1949 Aug 13;2(6572):276-8.

Jacobson JA, Danforth DN, Cowan KH, d'Angelo T, Steinberg SM, Pierce L, Lippman ME, Lichter AS, Glatstein E, Okunieff P. Ten-year results of a comparison of conservation with mastectomy in the treatment of stage I and II breast cancer. *N. Engl. J. Med.* 1995 Apr 6;332(14):907-11.

Jatoi I. Breast cancer: a systemic or local disease? *Am. J. Clin. Oncol.* 1997 Oct;20(5):536-9.

Kuerer HM, Newman LA. Lymphatic mapping and sentinel lymph node biopsy for breast cancer: developments and resolving controversies. *J. Clin.Oncol.* 2005 Mar 10;23(8):1698-705.

Lacour J, Le M, Caceres E, Koszarowski T, Veronesi U, Hill C. Radical mastectomy versus radical mastectomy plus internal mammary dissection. Ten year results of an international cooperative trial in breast cancer. *Cancer.* 1983 May 15;51(10):1941-3.

Lacour J, Lê MG, Hill C, Kramar A, Contesso G, Sarrazin D. Is it useful to remove internal mammary nodes in operable breast cancer? *Eur. J. Surg. Oncol.* 1987 Aug;13(4):309-14.

Lichter AS, Lippman ME, Danforth DN Jr, d'Angelo T, Steinberg SM, deMoss E, MacDonald HD, Reichert CM, Merino M, Swain SM, et al. Mastectomy versus breast-conserving therapy in the treatment of stage I and II carcinoma of the breast: a randomized trial at the National Cancer Institute. *J. Clin. Oncol.* 1992 Jun;10(6):976-83.

MacDonald I. Biological predeterminism in human cancer. *Surg. Gynecol. Obstet.* 1951 Apr;92(4):443-52.

Madden JL. Modified radical mastectomy. *Surg. Gynecol. Obstet.* 1965 Dec;121(6):1221-30.

Mansel RE, Fallowfield L, Kissin M, Goyal A, Newcombe RG, Dixon JM, Yiangou C, Horgan K, Bundred N, Monypenny I, England D, Sibbering M, Abdullah TI, Barr L, Chetty U, Sinnett DH, Fleissig A, Clarke D, Ell PJ. Randomized multicenter trial of sentinel node biopsy versus standard axillary treatment in operable breast cancer: the ALMANAC Trial. *J. Natl. Cancer Inst.* 2006 May 3;98(9):599-609.

Margottini M. Recent developments in the surgical treatment of breast carcinoma. *Acta Unio Int. Contra. Cancrum.* 1952;8(1):176-8.

Margottini M. Arguments in favour of super radical operations for carcinoma of the breast. *Acta Unio Int. Contra. Cancrum.* 1959;15:1037-9.

Meyer W. An improved method of the radical operation for carcinoma of the breast. *Med. Record* 1894;46: 746–9.

National Institutes of Health Consensus Development Panel. Treatment of early-stage breast cancer. *J. Natl. Cancer Inst. Monogr* 1992;11:137–42.

Park WW, Lees JC. The absolute curability of cancer of the breast. *Surg Gynecol. Obstet.* 1951 Aug;93(2):129-52.

Patey DH, Dyson WH. The prognosis of carcinoma of the breast in relation to the type of operation performed. *Br. J. Cancer.* 1948 Mar;2(1):7-13.

Sarrazin D, Lê MG, Arriagada R, Contesso G, Fontaine F, Spielmann M, Rochard F, Le Chevalier T, Lacour J. Ten-year results of a randomized trial comparing a conservative treatment to mastectomy in early breast cancer. *Radiother. Oncol.* 1989 Mar;14(3):177-84.

Straus K, Lichter A, Lippman M, Danforth D, Swain S, Cowan K, deMoss E, MacDonald H, Steinberg S, d'Angelo T, et al. Results of the National Cancer Institute early breast cancer trial. *J. Natl. Cancer Inst. Monogr.* 1992;(11):27-32.

Sugarbaker ED. Radical mastectomy combined with in-continuity resection of the homolateral internal mammary node chain. *Cancer.* 1953 Sep;6(5):969-79.

Urban JA. Surgical excision of internal mammary nodes for breast cancer. *Br. J. Surg.* 1964;51:209–12.

van Dongen JA, Voogd AC, Fentiman IS, Legrand C, Sylvester RJ, Tong D, van der Schueren E, Helle PA, van Zijl K, Bartelink H. Long-term results of a randomized trial comparing breast-conserving therapy with mastectomy: European Organization for Research and Treatment of Cancer 10801 trial. *J. Natl. Cancer Inst.* 2000 Jul 19;92(14):1143-50.

Verkooijen HM, Peeters PH, Pijnappel RM, Koot VC, Schipper ME, Borel Rinkes IH. Diagnostic accuracy of needle-localized open breast biopsy for impalpable breast disease. *Br. J. Surg.* 2000 Mar;87(3):344-7.

Veronesi U, Valagussa P. Inefficacy of internal mammary nodes dissection in breast cancer surgery. *Cancer.* 1981 Jan 1;47(1):170-5.

Veronesi U, Saccozzi R, Del Vecchio M, Banfi A, Clemente C, De Lena M, Gallus G, Greco M, Luini A, Marubini E, Muscolino G, Rilke F, Salvadori B, Zecchini A, Zucali R. Comparing radical mastectomy with quadrantectomy, axillary dissection, and radiotherapy in patients with small cancers of the breast. *N. Engl. J. Med.* 1981 Jul 2;305(1):6-11.

Veronesi U, Cascinelli N, Mariani L, Greco M, Saccozzi R, Luini A, Aguilar M, Marubini E. Twenty-year follow-up of a randomized study comparing breast-conserving surgery with radical mastectomy for early breast cancer. *N. Engl. J. Med.* 2002 Oct 17;347(16):1227-32.

Vlastos G, Verkooijen HM. Minimally invasive approaches for diagnosis and treatment of early-stage breast cancer. Oncologist. 2007 Jan;12(1):1-10.

Wangensteen OH. Another look at the super-radical operation for breast cancer. *Surgery.* 1957 May;41(5):857-61.

Wells CA. Quality assurance in breast cancer screening cytology: a review of the literature and a report on the U.K. national cytology scheme. *Eur. J. Cancer.* 1995;31A(2):273-80.

Chapter 5

Twentieth Century and Beyond Breast Cancer Radiotherapy

Abstract

X-rays were already used in breast cancer patients around 1900, and promising results were reported during the first half of the 20th century. However, the modern era of radiotherapy started in the 1950's, with the introduction of Cobalt-60 units and linear accelerators.With the decline of radical mastectomy, and on the basis of a wide series of clinical trials, radiotherapy was increasingly used to accompany simple mastectomy and, in more recent years, breast-conserving surgery. Whole-breast radiotherapy given for 5-7 weeks tends to be replaced by accelerated partial-breast radiotherapy given during less than 1 week. This latter includes interstitial and intracavitary brachytherapy, intraoperative radiation therapy and external beam accelerated therapy.

It is usually admitted, although still disputed [Leszczynski and Boyko 1997], that, in 1896, Emil *Herman* Grubbé (1875-1960) was the first to treat a patient with locally advanced breast cancer, Rose Lee, with radiation (reviewed in [Hodges 1964]). X-ray tube was placed in direct contact with the lesion. Nineteen one-hour radiation episodes were administered. Grubbé reported marked tumor regression, indicating that "radiotherapy" worked to some extent. However, Mrs Lee died two months later.

In 1897, Hermann *Moritz* Gocht (1869–1938) introduced the use of radiation for relief of pain in a case of breast carcinoma [Gocht 1897]. There was progressive improvement in radiotherapy technique into the mid-20th century.

It was soon apparent that X-ray exposure sometimes produced severe side effects, including burns and even cancer itself.In 1902 was reported the first case of radiation-induced cancer, a squamous cell carcinoma on the hand of an X-ray technician [Frieben 1902]. Within a decade, many more physicians and scientists, unaware of the dangers of radiation and of its health consequences, developed a variety of cancers. For instance Emil Grubbé's left hand was amputated in 1929; he subsequently underwent surgery for skin cancer, and died in 1960 from squamous cell carcinoma that had metastasized. The recognition of X-ray-associated dangers led to the development of more powerful and safer machines that delivered radiation by external beam. The other major alternative to surgery was radium implantation.

Between 1904 and 1906, French radiologist Jean *Alban* Bergonié (1857-1925) and histologist Louis Tribondeau (1872-1918) showed that cancer cells are more sensitive to X-rays than healthy cells, thus providing the first biological basis for radiation therapy utilizing X-rays. According to the "Bergonié-Tribondeau law", the radiosensitivity of a tissue depends on the number of undifferentiated cells in the tissue, their mitotic activity, and the length of time they are actively proliferating [Bergonié and Tribondeau 1906]. Like Grubbé, Bergonié died in 1925 from cancer caused by his research with X-rays.

In 1907, Albert *John* Ochsner (1858-1925) reported the use of post-mastectomy radiotherapy to control residual disease, with some apparent success [Ochsner 1907].

The growing enthusiasm for X-rays and radium as possible alternatives or supplements to surgery assumed major importance. By 1914, virtually every European capital had a radium institute, with the first being proposed in Paris around 1906.

In 1927, William *Sampson* Handley (1872-1962) had advocated treatment of involved internal mammary nodes with interstitial radium tubes [Handley 1927]. This line of study was extended by his son, Richard *Sampson* Handley (1909-1984), who routinely biopsied internal mammary lymph nodes during the performance of a radical mastectomy in a series of 119 patients and found metastases in 34% of patients.

An early detailed account of the use of local radium treatment in breast cancer patients was given by Stanford Cade (1895-1973) in his 1929 book "Radium Treatment of Cancer".

In 1929, *William* Roy Ward(1900-1982) reported on the use of external radium to treat 633 breast cancer patients during the period 1919-1927 [Ward 1929]. In every case, the disease had extended to tissues outside the breast itself. In these patients with advanced disease, results were judged encouraging, as about 40% of patients showed temporary benefit, even though they succumbed within three years of treatment. Ward stated that there were reasons for supposing that many local carcinoma recurrences could be prevented if pre-and postoperative radiotherapy were used more often. He also pointed out that recurrent disease after prophylactic radiation is very refractory to further radiotherapy and furthermore that a second treatment of any neoplasm is less effective than the primary treatment.

Geoffrey *Langdon* Keynes (1887-1982) began treating breast cancer with local irradiation in the 1920's. After tumor excision, interstitial radium needles were inserted throughout the breast, axilla, supraclavicular fossa and the upper three intercostal spaces. Five-year survival was 71% in patients (n=85) with stage I disease and 29% in patients (n=91) with stage II disease. These results appeared to be as good as those achieved by radical mastectomy. In 1927, Keynes abandoned the accepted operation of radical mastectomy and either conserved the breast or, for large tumors performed a simple mastectomy [Keynes 1932]. In the 1930's, Keynes became the most vocal critic of radical mastectomy, highlighting horrific disfigurement caused by the procedure.

He publically advocated breast conservation with ipsilateral radiation as treatment for cancer of the breast [Keynes 1937], but, as the sole practitioner of his method, he was criticized and his pioneer work did not receive wide approval. His method lapsed, especially after new techniques were developed with radiation apparatus that could deliver radiation from an external source. Other reasons were the limited availability of radium, handling problems, and fibrosis resulting from inaccuracies of dosage, and the Second World War.

In 1930, British surgeon George *Lenthal* Cheatle (1865-1951) suggested that a combination of external radiation followed by interstitial radium implant might be a useful treatment for primary breast cancer [Cheatle 1930].

In 1931, George *Edward* Pfahler (1874–1957) introduced postoperative radiation as routine treatment, improving the 5-year survival period for stage II breast cancer [Pfahler and Parry 1931]. Pfahler [Pfahler 1932] in the USA and Sakari Mustakallio (1899-1989) [Mustakallio 1945] in Finland reported series of 1022 and 701 patients, respectively, with breast cancer given external radiotherapy. These patients either were too frail or refused radical surgery. Results supported the view that the judicious use of radiotherapy could be as effective as radical surgery, while being considerably less harmful. For instance, Pfahler observed that the 5-year survival of patients with early disease was 80% and even patients with stage II disease fared better than historical controls. On the other hand, Muskatallio suggested that high doses of radiotherapy should be avoided, because they also have a detrimental effect.

Cobalt-60 was introduced in the 1950's as a radium substitute in teletherapy. The first cobalt-60 unit was installed in early 1951 at the Saskatoon Cancer Clinic in Canada. The conversion of stable cobalt-59 into the unstable cobalt-60 is accompanied by the emission of γ-rays, as it decays to nickel-60. These γ-rays are identical to X-rays, except in their origin. Cobalt-60 units may deliver energies higher than 1 million electron volts (MeV). The modern era of external beam therapy began. Cobalt-60 teletherapy was widely used to treat breast cancer since the 1960's. The simplicity of cobalt units give them the advantage of reduced maintenance, running costs and downtime when compared with linear accelerators.

First use of linear accelerator, or "linac" was made in 1954. The linac uses microwave energy to accelerate electrons to nearly the speed of light. As they reach maximum speed, the electrons collide with a metal target and release X-rays. Linear accelerators may deliver typical energies used range from 6 to 18 MeV

Comparison Radical Mastectomy vs. Simple Mastectomy + Radiation

After World War II, the Scottish Robert McWhirter (1904-1994) in Edinburgh, remembering Geoffrey Keynes' ideas, advocated simple mastectomy and high-voltage X-ray therapy to the internal mammary lymph nodes in the treatment of primary breast cancer. During a simple mastectomy, only the breast tissue and overlying skin are removed. The chest remains intact as does the axilla. The surgery is often accompanied by adjuvant radiotherapy. Unlike a radical mastectomy, a simple mastectomy leaves no cosmetic deformity of the chest wall. In 1948, McWhirter published a paper reporting on nearly 2,000 patients [McWhirter 1948] and showing improved survival rates with radiotherapy compared with radical surgery. McWhirter went on to accuse surgeons of selecting favorable cases when producing their follow-up results. Much of McWhirter's earlier work was confirmed in 1959 by the randomized study of English radiologist James *Ralston Kennedy* Paterson (1897 - 1981) and statistician Marion *Howard* Russell (1907-1966) at the Christie Hospital in Manchester (UK) on 1461 patients, entered between 1949 and 1955, with a minimum follow-up of 4 years [Paterson and Russell 1959]. McWhirter undoubtedly laid the foundations for the eventual use of radiotherapy in breast-conserving surgery. Surgery was the sole treatment approach to breast cancer for over half of the 20th century, but the trend towards minimization of surgery supplemented by radiation therapy had begun.

A number of clinical trials confirmed McWhirter's observations. For instance, in 1954, Mustakallio reported that removing only the breast and irradiating suspicious lymph nodes in order to destroy any remaining cancer showed results comparable to those obtained by radical mastectomy [Mustakallio 1954]. From 1951 to 1957, a prospective clinical trial was carried out in Copenhagen by Sigvard Kaae (1913-2001) and Helge Johansen. The results of extended radical mastectomy (removal of the breast, chest muscles, axillary, supraclavicular, and internal mammary nodes) without postoperative radiation were compared with simple mastectomy with postoperative radiation. The 5-year study included 206 patients from the extended radical group and 209 from the simple mastectomy. The overall survival and recurrence rates at 5- and 10-year intervals were similar with both treatments.

Comparison Radical or Simple Mastectomy vs. Lumpectomy, Tylectomy, Quadrantectomy + Radiation (Breast-Conserving Therapy)

Since the 1950's, radical mastectomy was "in concurrence" not only with simple mastectomy followed by local radiotherapy, but also, increasingly, with local tumor excision (variously known as tylectomy, lumpectomy or quadrantectomy) followed by local radiotherapy. This less-disfiguring operation was practiced by pioneers such as Sakari Mustakallio [Mustakallio 1954; work reviewed in [Sakari Mustakallio Centennial Symposium 1999]), François Baclesse (1896-1967) [Baclesse 1960], Leslie Wise [Wise et al. 1971] and many others, who have produced end-results that were no worse than the more extensive classical surgical procedures.

In the 1980's and 1990's, a series of retrospective studies and of prospective randomized clinical trials (see chapter 4) have established breast-conserving therapy as the preferred treatment of early stages (stages I and II) breast cancer, as compared to radical mastectomy.

During the 1990's, breast-conserving therapy was found to result in survival equivalent to that achieved with mastectomy, among patients with early-stage breast cancer, in six prospective randomized trials as well as in multiple retrospective studies in the United States and Europe [Fourquet *et al.* 1989; Fowble *et al.* 1990 ; Sarrazin e*t al.* 1990 ; Kurtz *et al.* 1990 ; Veronesi *et al.* 1990 ; Blichert-Toft *et al.* 1992; van Dongen *et al.* 1992 ; Fisher *et al.* 1995; Gage *et al.* 1995 ; Jacobson *et al.* 1995]

Comparison Lumpectomy, Tylectomy vs. Lumpectomy, Tylectomy + Radiation

Several clinical trials have demonstrated that the addition of irradiation to wide excision in early breast cancers significantly reduced the risk of breast recurrence when compared with wide excision alone (see for instance [Fisher *et al.* 1989, Clark *et al.* 1992, Veronesi *et al.* 1993]).

In 2003,a systematic review of radiation therapy trials in breast cancer was done, based on data from 29 randomized trials, 6 meta-analyses and 5 retrospective studies. In total, 40 scientific articles were included, involving 41 204 patients. It was concluded that:

- There is strong evidence for a substantial reduction in locoregional recurrence rate following postmastectomy radiation therapy to the chest wall and the regional nodal areas.
- There is strong evidence that postmastectomy radiation therapy increases the disease-free survival rate.
- There are conflicting data regarding the impact of postmastectomy radiotherapy upon overall survival.
- There is strong evidence that breast cancer specific survival is improved by postmastectomy radiotherapy.
- There is strong evidence for a decrease in non-breast cancer specific survival after postmastectomy radiotherapy.
- There is some evidence that overall survival is increased by optimal postmastectomy radiation therapy.
- There is strong evidence that postmastectomy radiotherapy in addition to surgery and systemic therapy in mainly node-positive patients decreases local recurrence rate and improves survival.

- There is moderate evidence that the decrease in non-breast cancer specific survival is attributed to cardiovascular disease in irradiated patients.
- There are conflicting data whether breast conservation surgery plus radiotherapy is comparable to modified radical mastectomy alone in terms of local recurrence rate.
- There is strong evidence that breast conservation surgery plus radiotherapy is comparable to modified radical mastectomy alone in terms of disease-free survival and overall survival.
- There is strong evidence that postoperative radiotherapy to the breast following breast conservation surgery results in a statistically and clinically significant reduction of ipsilateral breast recurrences followed by diminished need for salvage mastectomies.
- There is strong evidence that the omission of postoperative radiotherapy to the breast following breast conservation surgery has no impact on overall survival. In one meta-analysis including three randomized studies a survival advantage is demonstrated by Bayesian statistics.
- There is strong evidence that the addition of a radiation boost after conventional radiotherapy to the tumor bed after breast conservation surgery significantly decreases the risk of ipsilateral breast recurrences but has no impact on overall survival after short follow-up.
- There is strong evidence for the use of postoperative radiotherapy to the breast following breast conservation surgery for DCIS (ductal breast cancer in situ). Radiotherapy leads to a clinically and statistically significant reduction of both non-invasive and invasive ipsilateral breast recurrences [Rutqvist et al. 2003].

In 2005, in an overview of randomized trials comparing radiotherapy vs. no radiotherapy and involving a total of 23,500 early breast cancer patients, radiotherapy was seen to produce similar proportional reductions in local recurrence in all women (irrespective of age or tumor characteristics) and in all major trials of radiotherapy versus not (recent or older; with or without systemic therapy). There was, at least with some of the older radiotherapy regimens, a significant excess incidence of contralateral breast cancer and a significant excess of non-breast-cancer mortality in irradiated women. Both were slight during the first 5 years, but continued after year 15. The excess mortality was mainly from heart disease and lung cancer [Clarke *et al.* 2005].

Whole-Breast vs. Partial Breast Radiation Therapy

Conventional radiation therapy (RT) after breast-conserving surgery consists of 5-7 weeks of external-beam RT (ERT) of the whole breast ("whole-breast RT", or WBRT). In ERT, as the name implies, the high-energy X-rays beam is generated outside the patient (usually by a linear accelerator). Despite the undisputed efficacy of this treatment approach, the necessity of electively treating the entire breast for presumed occult disease is uncertain. Various ways to confine radiotherapy to the tumor bed in accelerated fractionation schemes have been evaluated in many studies.These methods are known as "partial breast RT" (PBRT) or "partial breast irradiation" (PBI) and they have generally shown equivalence with traditional WBRI.The major advantage of PBI is the time compression of treatment down to less than 1 week compared with 5-7 weeks for WBRT [Chen and Vicini 2007; Swanson and Vicini 2008]. It is the reason why the term of "accelerated PBI", or APBI is also frequently used.

A variety of APBI techniques are currently available, including:

A. interstitial brachytherapy
B. intraoperative radiation therapy (IORT)
C. intracavitary brachytherapy
D. external beam (EB)-APBI, itself including:
    –   3D-CRT
    –   IMRT
    –   helical tomotherapy
    –   PBRT

In the late 1970's, interstitial radiotherapy (or brachytherapy) for breast cancer was (re)introduced. Brachytherapy is a type of radiotherapy in which the radiation source is placed within or close to the target site, using multicatheter devices. This contrasts with external-beam radiotherapy (teletherapy), in which the radiation source is generally 80—100 cm away from the patient.

A form of brachytherapy had been performed by William Handley as early as in 1922, using radium (see above). This technique was revived following the introduction of isotopes such as Cesium (Cs)-137 and Iridium (Ir)-192, which have shorter half-lives than radium and can be shielded more easily because of their lower energies. Also determinant were the availability of computerized dosimetry and the refinement of implantation techniques [Goffinet *et al.* 1980].

Although both low-dose–rate (LDR) and high-dose-rate (HDR) brachytherapy have been used in breast cancer patients, LDR has now largely been abandoned in favor of the most convenient outpatient-based HDR approach that better controls the dose delivery and radiation safety concerns of LDR. The most widely used HDR source is Ir-192. This isotope has a dose rate of about 100 cGy/min.

Brachytherapy was progressively improved through the addition of image guidance and the availability of 3D-treatment planning for brachytherapy [Das *et al.* 2004].

A) In the late 1980's, intraoperative electron beam breast cancer therapy (intraoperative radiation therapy, or IORT) was introduced [Dobelbower *et al.* 1989]. Electron beams are produced by linear accelerators and delivered when patients are still in surgery. Randomized trials comparing IORT with postoperative radiation in terms of local recurrence, cosmesis, or local toxicity, are ongoing [Skandarajah *et al.* 2009]. Of note, another type of IORT is high-dose rate (HDR)-brachytherapy. IORT is sometimes referred to as IntraOperative Electron Radiation Therapy (IOERT).

B) Since 2002, intracavitary brachytherapy is illustrated by the MammoSite radiotherapy system [Keisch *et al.* 2003]. It is an alternative to interstitial brachytherapy with either seeds or needles to treat the intact breast lumpectomy site.In intracavitary brachytherapy, which was developed in an attempt to simplify the APBI implantation process, the lumpectomy cavity is dilated by a balloon and a single high-dose radiation source is positioned within the central portion of the balloon to deliver a uniform dose to the walls of the lumpectomy cavity.The primary justification for breast brachytherapy is a lack of patient compliance with conventional post-operative external beam radiotherapy.As compared to 5-7 weeks of external beam therapy, the MammoSite system offers the convenience of a short course of treatment, usually 10 twice-daily HDR applications over 5 days.Additional methods of balloon brachytherapy, including Xoft and SenoRx Contura have been developed [Strauss and Dickler 2009].

C) In the early 2000's, four "external beam accelerated partial breast irradiation" (EB-APBI) techniques have been introduced:

Three-dimensional conformal radiotherapy (3D-CRT) [Baglan *et al.* 2003] uses CT or MRI simulation images to create a three-dimensional target. As compared to conventional external beam radiotherapy, it thus uses three parameters (width, height and depth) instead of the traditional two (width and height) to improve the precision. Breast tumor receives a relatively homogenous and high radiation dose while surrounding normal breast tissue receives a relatively lower dose.Intensity-modulated radiation therapy (IMRT, reviewed in [Sanghani and Mignano 2006]). In conventional radiation treatments, uniform radiation doses are delivered to large regions of tissue. In IMRT, which is in fact an enhanced form of 3D-CRT, a multi-leaf collimator moves dynamically to generate radiation beams of varying intensities. These simultaneously deliver different doses of radiation to small areas of tissue, more intensely on tumor deposits and in limited dose to nearly normal tissues. Helical tomotherapy uses a combination of a linear accelerator and a helical CT scanner, for the purpose of rotational delivery of IMRT. The imaging capacity conferred by the CT component allows targeted regions to be visualized prior to, during, and immediately after each treatment.Proton beam radiation therapy (PBRT). Compared with traditional radiation therapy with photons or electrons, PBRT offers a more precise dose distribution. Several studies have shown that cardiac mortality due to acute myocardial ischemia can increase for left-sided breast cancer patients treated with three-dimensional (3D) planning because of the exposure of a portion of the left ventricle to high radiation doses [Roychoudhuri *et al.* 2007]. The effect of PBRT on the tumor is likely to be the same with protons as with photons or electrons, but the dose in sensitive tissues in the heart and the lung may be reduced considerably, so that very low toxicity can be expected to develop later. Breast cancer is a potential target for proton therapy, in particular for patients with left-sided breast cancer [Lomax *et al.* 2003].

References

Baclesse F, Ennuyer A, Cheguillaume J. [May a simple tumorectomy followed by radiotherapy be performed in the case of mammary tumor?] *J. Radiol. Electrol. Med. Nucl.* 1960 Mar-Apr;41:137-9.

Baglan KL, Sharpe MB, Jaffray D, Frazier RC, Fayad J, Kestin LL, Remouchamps V, Martinez AA, Wong J, Vicini FA. Accelerated partial breast irradiation using 3D conformal radiation therapy (3D-CRT). *Int. J.Radiat. Oncol. Biol. Phys.* 2003 Feb 1;55(2):302-11.

Bergonié J, Tribondeau L. Interprétation de quelques résultats de la radiothérapie et essai de fixation d'une technique rationnelle. Note présentée par d'Arsonval. [n.p.] 1906. Extract from Académie des sciences (France). Séance du 10 Décembre 1906.

Blichert-Toft M, Rose C, Andersen JA, Overgaard M, Axelsson CK, Andersen KW, Mouridsen HT. Danish randomized trial comparing breast conservation therapy with mastectomy: Six years of life-table analysis. *J. Natl. Cancer Inst. Monogr.* 1992;(11):19-25.

Cheatle L. A lecture on treatment of mammary carcinoma by radiation. *Br. Med. J.* 1930;1:807-11.

Chen PY, Vicini FA. Partial breast irradiation. Patient selection, guidelines for treatment, and current results. Front Radiat Ther Oncol. 2007;40:253-71.

Clark RM, McCulloch PB, Levine MN, Lipa M, Wilkinson RH, Mahoney LJ, Basrur VR, Nair BD, McDermot RS, Wong CS, Corbett PJ. Randomized clinical trial to assess the effectiveness of breast irradiation following lumpectomy and axillary dissection for node-negative breast cancer. *J. Natl. Cancer Inst.* 1992 May 6;84(9):683-9.

Clarke M, Collins R, Darby S, Davies C, Elphinstone P, Evans E, Godwin J, Gray R, Hicks C, James S, MacKinnon E, McGale P, McHugh T, Peto R, Taylor C, Wang Y; Early Breast Cancer Trialists' Collaborative Group (EBCTCG). Effects of radiotherapy and of differences in the extent of surgery for early breast cancer on local recurrence and 15-year survival: an overview of the randomised trials. *Lancet.* 2005 Dec 17;366(9503):2087-106.

Das RK, Patel R, Shah H, Odau H, Kuske RR. 3D CT-based high-dose-rate breast brachytherapy implants: treatment planning and quality assurance. *Int. J. Radiat. Oncol. Biol. Phys.* 2004 Jul 15;59(4):1224-8.

Dobelbower RR, Merrick HW, Eltaki A, Bronn DG. Intraoperative electron beam therapy and external photon beam therapy with lumpectomy as primary treatment for early breast cancer. *Ann. Radiol.* (Paris). 1989;32(6):497-501.

Fisher B, Redmond C, Poisson R, et al. Eight-year results of a randomized clinical trial comparing total mastectomy and lumpectomy with or without irradiation in the treatment of breast cancer. *N. Engl. J. Med.* 1989;320:822-8.

Fisher B, Anderson S, Redmond CK, Wolmark N, Wickerham DL, Cronin WM. Reanalysis and results after 12 years of follow-up in a randomized clinical trial comparing total mastectomy with lumpectomy with or without irradiation in the treatment of breast cancer. *N. Engl. J. Med.* 1995 Nov 30;333(22):1456-61.

Fowble B, Solin LJ, Schultz DJ, Rubenstein J, Goodman RL. Breast recurrence following conservative surgery and radiation: Patterns of failure, prognosis, and pathologic findings from mastectomy specimens with implications for treatment. *Int. J. Radiat. Oncol. Biol. Phys.* 1990 Oct;19(4):833-42.

Fourquet A, Campana F, Zafrani B, Mosseri V, Vielh P, Durand JC, Vilcoq JR. Prognostic factors of breast recurrence in the conservative management of early breast cancer: A 25-year follow-up. *Int. J. Radiat. Oncol. Biol. Phys.* 1989 Oct;17(4):719-25.

Frieben H. Demonstration eines Cancroïd des rechten Handrückens, das sich nach langedaurnder Einwirkung von Röntgenstrahlen entwickelt hatte. Forsch Röntgenstr. 1902;6:106.

Gage I, Recht A, Gelman R, Nixon AJ, Silver B, Bornstein BA, Harris JR. Long-term outcome following breast-conserving surgery and radiation therapy. *Int. J. Radiat. Oncol. Biol. Phys.* 1995 Sep 30;33(2):245-51.

Gocht HM. Therapeutische Verwendung der Röntgenstahlen. Fortschr Geb Rontgenstr. 1897-1898;I:14-22.

Goffinet DR, Martinez A, Pooler D, Palos B, Cox R. Brachytherapy renaissance. *Front Radiat. Ther. Oncol.* 1980;15:43-57.

Handley WS. Parasternal invasion of the thorax in breast cancer and its suppression by the use of radium tubes as an operative precaution. *Surg. Gynec. and Obstet.* 1927;45:721–8.

Hodges PC. Dr. Emil H. Grubbe, pioneer Chicago radiologist. *Postgrad. Med.* 1964 Jun;35:A85-7.

Jacobson JA, Danforth DN, Cowan KH, d'Angelo T, Steinberg SM, Pierce L, Lippman ME, Lichter AS, Glatstein E, Okunieff P. Ten-year results f a comparison of conservation surgery with mastectomy in the reatment of stage I and II breast cancer. *N. Engl. J. Med.* 1995 Apr 6;332(14):907-11.

Keisch M, Vicini F, Kuske RR, Hebert M, White J, Quiet C, Arthur D, Scroggins T, Streeter O. Initial clinical experience with the MammoSite breast brachytherapy applicator in women with early-stage breast cancer treated with breast-conserving therapy. *Int. J. Radiat. Oncol. Biol. Phys.* 2003 Feb 1;55(2):289-93.

Keynes GL. The radium treatment of carcinoma of the breast. *Br. J. Surg.* 1932;19:415–80.

Keynes GL. The place of radium in the treatment of cancer of the breast. *Ann. Surg.* 1937 Oct;106(4):619-30.

Kurtz JM, Spitalier JM, Amalric R, Brandone H, Ayme Y, Jacquemier J, Hans D, Bressac C. The prognostic ignificance of late local recurrence after breast-conserving therapy. *Int. J. Radiat. Oncol. Biol. Phys.* 1990 Jan;18(1):87-93.

Leszczynski K, Boyko S. On the controversies surrounding the origins of radiation therapy. *Radiother. Oncol.* 1997 Mar;42(3):213-7.

Lomax AJ, Cella L, Weber D, Kurtz JM, Miralbell R. Potential role of intensity-modulated photons and protons in the treatment of the breast and regional nodes. *Int. J. Radiat. Oncol. Biol. Phys.* 2003;55:785–92.

McWhirter R. The value of simple mastectomy and radiotherapy in the treatment of cancer of the breast. Br J Radiol. 1948 Dec;21(252):599-610.

Mustakallio S. Uber die Möglichkeiten der Rontgentherapie bei der Behandlung des Brustkrebses. *Acta Radiol.* 1945;26:503-11.

Mustakallio S. Treatment of breast cancer by tumor extirpation and roentgen therapy instead of radical operation. *J. Fac. Radio.* 1954;6:23-6.

Ochsner A 3rd. Final Results in 164 Cases of Carcinoma of the Breast Operated upon during the Past Fourteen Years at the Augustana Hospital 1907 *Ann. Surg.* 1907 July;46(1):28–42.

Paterson R, Russell MH. Breast cancer: evaluation of post-operative radiotherapy. *J. Fac. Radiol.* 1959;10:174–80.

Pfahler GE, Parry LD. Rontgen therapy in carcinoma of the breast: a statistical study of 977 private cases. *Ann. Surg* 1931;93:412–27.

Pfahler GE. Results of radiation therapy in 1022 private cases of carcinoma of the breast from 1902 to 1928. *Am. J. Roentgenol. Rad. Ther.* 1932;27:497-508.

Roychoudhuri R, Robinson D, Putcha V, Cuzick J, Darby S, Møller H. Increased cardiovascular mortality more than fifteen years after radiotherapy for breast cancer: A population-based study. *BMC Cancer.* 2007 Jan 15;7:9.

Rutqvist LE, Rose C, Cavallin-Ståhl E. A systematic overview of radiation therapy effects in breast cancer. *Acta Oncol.* 2003;42(5-6):532-45.

Sakari Mustakallio Centennial Symposium. Helsinki, Finland, 8-9 January 1999. Proceedings. [No authors listed] *Acta Oncol.* 1999;38 Suppl 13:1-83.

Sanghani M, Mignano J. Intensity modulated radiation therapy: a review of current practice and future directions. *Technol. Cancer Res. Treat.* 2006 Oct;5(5):447-50.

Sarrazin D, Lê MG, Arriagada R, Contesso G, Fontaine F, Spielmann M, Rochard F, Le Chevalier T, Lacour J. Ten-year results of a randomized trial comparing a conservative treatment to mastectomy in early breast cancer. *Radiother Oncol.* 1989 Mar;14(3):177-84.

Skandarajah AR, Lynch AC, Mackay JR, Ngan S, Heriot AG. The role of intraoperative radiotherapy in solid tumors. *Ann. Surg. Oncol.* 2009 Mar;16(3):735-44.

Strauss JB, Dickler A. Accelerated partial breast irradiation utilizing balloon brachytherapy techniques. *Radiother Oncol.* 2009 May;91(2):157-65.

Swanson TA, Vicini FA. Overview of accelerated partial breast irradiation. *Curr. Oncol. Rep.* 2008 Jan;10(1):54-60.

van Dongen JA, Bartelink H, Fentiman IS, Lerut T, Mignolet F, Olthuis G, van der Schueren E, Sylvester R, Winter J, van Zijl K. Randomized clinical trial to assess the value of breast-conserving therapy in stage I and II breast cancer, EORTC 10801 trial. *J. Natl. Cancer Inst. Monogr.* 1992;(11):15-8.

Veronesi U, Salvadori B, Luini A, Banfi A, Zucali R, Del Vecchio M, Saccozzi R, Beretta E, Boracchi P, Farante G, et al. Conservative treatment of early breast cancer: Long-term results of 1232 cases treated with quadrantectomy, axillary dissection, and radiotherapy. *Ann. Surg.* 1990 Mar;211(3):250-9.

Veronesi U, Luini A, Del Vecchio M, Greco M, Galimberti V, Merson M, Rilke F, Sacchini V, Saccozzi R, Savio T, Zucali R, Zurrida S, Salvadori B. Radiotherapy after breast-preserving surgery in women with localized cancer of the breast. *N. Engl. J. Med.* 1993 Jun 3;328(22):1587-91.

Ward R. Inoperable carcinoma of the breast treated with radium. *Br. Med. J.* 1929;1:242-4.

Wise L, Mason AY, Ackerman LV. Local excision and irradiation: an alternative method for the treatment of early mammary cancer. *Ann. Surg.* 1971 Sep;174(3):392-401.

Chapter 6

Twentieth Century and Beyond Breast Cancer Chemotherapy

Abstract

Although the concept was born around 1900, it was not before the 1940's that the era of chemotherapy really started. Some compounds introduced in the 1950's, such as fluorouracil and cyclophosphamide, are still used in breast cancer patients. More recently introduced therapeutic molecules include the anthracyclines (doxorubicin and epirubicin), the antimetabolites (capecitabine and gemcitabine) and the taxanes (paclitaxel and docetaxel). Heterogeneity of breast tumors led to the use of combination therapy, which has only partially overcome the barrier. The concepts of adjuvant (postoperative) and neoadjuvant (preoperative) therapies were introduced in the 1970's and 1980's, respectively. Metronomic chemotherapy was developed in the 2000's. Clinical trials continue to examine new molecules to improve chemotherapeutical control of tumor progression.

The term "chemotherapy" was introduced around 1900 and is usually attributed to the German chemist Paul Ehrlich (1854-1915). It was defined as "the controlled use of chemicals to treat disease" [De Vita and Chu 2008]. Paul Ehrlich was the first to show that animal models were effective to screen a series of chemicals for their potential activity against diseases, an accomplishment that had major ramifications for cancer drug development. Ehrlich, with colleagues, examined aniline dyes and arsenicals as possible treatments for diseases such as trypanosomiasis and syphilis. He also discovered the action of vinylamine, currently known as ethyleneimine, the first alkylating agent identified. Ehrlich proposed the idea that foreign microbes (and, by extension, cancer cells) might posses biochemically unique binding sites whose blockade (by "magic bullets", in german "Zauberkugel") could result in targeted destruction of the invading microbe (or cancer cell) without harm to healthy tissues [Strebhardt and Ullrich 2008].

It was not before the 1940's that the era of chemotherapy really started, and this was mainly a consequence of World War II. In 1946, in a landmark experiment, pharmacologists Louis *Sanford* Goodman (1906-2000) and Alfred Gilman (1908-1984), and surgeon Gustaf *Elmer* Lindskog (1903-2002) found that injections of mustine (a compound related to nitrogen mustard) caused a reduction in tumor size in a patient with lymphoma. However, the tumor slowly regenerated. A subsequent course of therapy resulted in only partial improvement and a third course had relatively little effect (see [Gilman and Philips 1946] and [Goodman *et al.* 1984]).

A few years later, in 1948, pediatric pathologist Sidney Farber (1903-1973) demonstrated that folic acid analogues ("antifolates"), such as aminopterin and amethopterin (methotrexate), induced remission in childhood acute leukaemia [Farber and Diamond 1948], but his observations met with disbelief. Methotrexate was FDA-approved as anticancer drug in 1953. Its effects on breast cancer were first reported in the first half of 1960's and the drug is still used in combination therapy for breast cancer today.

Throughout the 1940's and 1950's, various antifolates, antimetabolites and alkylating agents were studied and used to treat cancer. Chemotherapy became the cutting edge of cancer research. Unfortunately, despite the initial enthusiasm for these treatments, remissions generally turned out to be brief and incomplete.

In 1956, cyclophosphamide was synthesized by Herbert Arnold (1909-1973), Friedrich Bourseaux (b. 1918) and Norbert Brock (1912-2008) [Arnold *et al.* 1958]. This orally available nitrogen mustard (alkylating agent) was approved by FDA as anticancer drug in 1959. It has become the most-used of its class in breast cancer therapy.

In 1957, Charles Heidelberger (1920-1983) and colleagues discovered 5-fluorouracil (or fluorouracil), which was approved by FDA as anticancer drug in 1962. Fluorouracil, a pyrimidine analog, is still a key chemotherapy agent (antimetabolite) for treating breast cancer today [Heidelberger *et al.* 1957].

Still in 1957, Bernard Fisher set up the Surgical Adjuvant Chemotherapy Breast Project, which would later become the National Surgical Adjuvant Breast Project (NSABP) to study various aspects of breast cancer treatment.

The group began to question some of Halsted's principles and went on to reverse many of his theories.

The first randomized double blind clinical trial ("NSABP B01") evaluating the use of systemic therapy for the treatment of breast cancer was begun in 1958. At that time, researchers theorized that women died of breast cancer despite radical surgery because tumor cells were dislodged during the operation. It was believed that the dissemination of those cells resulted in metastasis and subsequent death. In the NSABP B01 study (data reported in [Noer 1963]), more than 800 women were treated with radical mastectomy either with or without perioperative triethylene-thiophosphoramide (thiotepa), an alkylating agent. Despite the fact that thiotepa was used in almost homeopathic doses, patients experienced some undesirable side effects that led surgeons to be reluctant about using such therapy. The study did, however, demonstrate for the first time that systemic therapy could perturb the natural history of women with breast cancer [Travis 2005].

By 1958, the first real cure of a disseminated tumor, choriocarcinoma, was reported [Li et al. 1958]. Young medical researcher Min Chiu Li (d. 1980), working with oncologist Roy Hertz (1909-2002), was thus the first to demonstrate that systemic chemotherapy with methotrexate alone could result in the cure of a widely metastatic malignant disease [Freireich 2002]. Despite this, Min Chiu Li was fired from the U.S. National Cancer Institute (NCI) for the sin of being too far ahead of his time. However, its work heralded the age of modern chemotherapy.

In 1963, Ezra Greenspan (1919-2004) published the results of a trial of methotrexate and thiotepa in women with metastatic breast and ovarian cancers. Greenspan is seen as the "Father of modern combination cancer chemotherapy".

In 1965, Emil Frei III (b. 1924), Emil "Jay" Freireich (b. 1927), James *Frederick* Holland (b. 1925) and colleagues used combination chemotherapy. They produced remissions in children with acute lymphoblastic leukaemia by administering methotrexate, vincristine, 6-mercaptopurine and prednisone (the "POMP regimen") [Frei et al. 1965]. This strategy of combining chemotherapy agents having different sites of action and non-overlapping toxicities was a major breakthrough and led to unrivaled success in the treatment of blood diseases such as leukemias and Hodgkin's disease in the 1960s and 1970s. Heterogeneity of the tumor cell population was identified as a major obstacle to the effectiveness of chemotherapy, and the combination drug approach, still used (with different drugs) in breast cancer management today, partially overcame this barrier. Investigators began to use combination chemotherapy in advanced breast cancer in the late 1960s with some encouraging results (see notably [Carbone 1975]).

In 1967, the taxane paclitaxel was discovered from the bark of the Pacific yew tree (*Taxus brevifolia*). The drug later became a key tool for the treatment of breast cancer (approved by FDA in 1994). Another widely used taxane, docetaxel, an esterified product of 10-deacetyl baccatin III and a semi-synthetic analogue of paclitaxel, was introduced in clinical trials in the 1990's.

The anthracycline doxorubicin was described in 1969 by Federico-*Maria* Arcamone (b. 1928) and colleagues. It was isolated from the microorganism*Streptomyces peucetius*. As this microorganism was obtained on the Adriatic coast of Italy, doxorubicin is also frequently named adriamycin [Arcamone *et al.* 1969]. Doxorubicin, approved by FDA in 1974, was rapidly introduced in breast cancer chemotherapy. It is still one of the most active agents against breast cancer. Epirubicin, another anthracycline widely used in breast cancer therapy, was synthesized in an effort to find agents with a superior therapeutic index to the parent compound doxorubicin [Ganzina 1983].

Mainly during the 1960's, Howard *Earle* Skipper (1915-2006) conducted a series of classic experiments using the L1210 mouse leukemia model. These experiments established that to cure L1210, it was necessary to eradicate the last leukemia cell because back extrapolations of survival after treatment suggested that one surviving cell was sufficient to kill a mouse [Skipper *et al.* 1964]. Skipper formulated a "cell kill law", stating that a given dose of drug killed a constant fraction of tumor cells not a constant number, regardless of the body burden of tumor cells. Therefore success of (combination) chemotherapy would depend on the number of cells present at the beginning of each treatment (see notably [Skipper 1979]).

The 1970's were characterized by the development of postoperative, or adjuvant, chemotherapy. This form of therapy was supported by the fact that a majority of patients with breast cancer presented with locoregional disease, of which most developed recurrences if only the best locoregional treatment was used.For those patients presenting with a high risk of relapse, it was thus tempting to use drugs effective in patients with advanced breast cancer. Moreover, Skipper's cell kill law, and the invariable inverse relation between cell number and curability, suggested that drugs effective against advanced disease might work better in the adjuvant situation with only micrometastases to deal with [Schabel 1975; Young and De Vita 1970].

The two "landmark" trials examining the use of adjuvant chemotherapy were started in the early 1970's.Bernard Fisher (1918-) and colleagues of the

National Surgical Adjuvant Breast Project (NSABP) tested alkylating agent melphalan (L-PAM, L-Sarcolysin Phenylalanine Mustard) in a randomized controlled trial. Gianni Bonadonna (b. 1934) of the Istituto Nazionale Tumori, in Milan, Italy along with Umberto Veronesi conducted a randomized controlled trial of a CMF (cyclophosphamide-methotrexate-5'fluorouracil) combination versus no therapy in patients with node-positive, operable breast cancer.

Within 5 years, both studies were complete and the L-PAM study was reported to much fanfare when published in the New England Journal of Medicine in 1975, simultaneous with the announcement that the wives of the USA President, Betty Ford, and the Vice President, Happy Rockefeller, were diagnosed with breast cancer [Fisher *et al.* 1975]. These data provided the initial evidence that adjuvant chemotherapy could alter the natural history of breast cancer and improve survival. The Bonadonna CMF study was published a year later [Bonadonna *et al.* 1976]. Both studies were positive, and the results set off a cascade of adjuvant studies in breast cancer, with exciting results that have contributed to the significant decline in mortality for breast cancer. Adjuvant CMF became the gold standard against which new drug regimens were tested. Today a significant majority of patients with invasive carcinomas measuring greater than 1 cm receives some form of adjuvant therapy.

First attempts to use preoperative adjuvant ("neoadjuvant") therapy in breast cancer patients were made in the first half of the 1980's (see for instance reviews by [Papaioannou 1985; Goldie 1985]). Neoadjuvant therapy has various advantages: systemic treatment as the initial attack against operable breast cancer may destroy clonogenic cells in the primary tumor which are responsible for the development of metastases; primary tumor shrinkage following neoadjuvant systemic therapy may serve as an early, simple, and inexpensive index of the overall chemosensitivity of the tumor; systemic treatment as soon as the diagnosis is made may prevent the development of drug-resistant mutations, which are likely to form spontaneously early in the natural history of the disease; the average delay of about 1 month in the treatment of micrometastases in the postoperative adjuvant setting leads to at least a 30% increase of micrometastatic tumor burden, which can be prevented by preoperative treatment (according to [Papaioannou 1985]).

The interest of neoadjuvant approach was established in the first half of 1990's, based on a series of randomized controlled studies in which patients were managed using either the adjuvant or neoadjuvant approaches (reviewed in [Aapro 2001])

During the 1980's, there was a trend to higher drug doses, and this led clinicians to experiment with doses of chemotherapy previously found to be lethal by harvesting patients' bone marrow before treatment and returning it afterwards. However, the findings of major randomized trials did not support the use of this therapy in patients with breast cancer (for more details on the "rise and fall" of high-dose therapy, see [Frei 1985] and the review of [Welch and Mogielnicki 2002]).

In the 1980's, the pharmaceutical industry screened more new compounds and researchers carried out elaborated trials with ever more complex combinations. New drugs introduced at that time and still used to treat breast cancer patients include the antimetabolites capecitabine and gemcitabine. There was a great hope that each breast tumor eventually would be cured. However, in the 1990's, initial optimism about combination chemotherapy as a cure-all for cancer, waned. Early dramatic successes with rare cancers such as acute lymphoblastic leukaemia did not translate to the more common cancers, such as breast cancer. At the same time, advances in molecular and genetic approaches to understanding the cell biology of cancer began to influence research and development [Leaf 2004]. Attention turned from chemotherapy to conventional drugs, such as antiestrogens and aromatase inhibitors, and to targeted therapies, such as monoclonal antibodies and small kinase inhibitors.

Metronomic chemotherapy was developed in the 2000's. In metronomic chemotherapy, low doses of chemotherapy drugs (each significantly below the maximum tolerated dose [MTD]) are given at frequent, even daily, intervals for extended periods with no prolonged drug-free intervals. The doses are low enough that even the cumulative dose may be lower than the MTD. These low doses result in reduced toxicity and a reduced reliance on growth factor support to recover from the myelosuppression. Metronomic chemotherapy was designed primarily to be antiangiogenic instead of cytotoxic. Chemotherapy drugs interfere with cell division and affect all dividing cells, including the endothelial cells involved with new blood vessel formation in the growing tumor. Usually, the damaged endothelial cells are repaired or replaced during the 3- to 4-week breaks normally used to recover from the side effects of chemotherapy [Browder 2000]. In metronomic chemotherapy, the use of very short cycles does not allow sufficient time for this to occur. In addition, because the endothelial cells are normal and genetically stable, they are unlikely to acquire drug resistance, a phenomenon that is common in genetically unstable tumor cells. They will continue to respond to the mitosis-inhibiting effects of the chemotherapy through repeated doses.

Initial studies have been promising, but these studies were very small. Larger controlled trials are needed to provide additional evidence for the clinical usefulness of metronomic chemotherapy [Singletary 2007]. Metronomic chemotherapy targets a different cell population than standard therapies, so it may be combined with other low-impact modalities, such as targeted therapies, endocrine therapy, or antitumor vaccines.

A significant drawback with chemotherapy is that because it also affects normal cells it has some serious and unpleasant side-effects (such as alopecia, impaired immunity, cardiotoxicity). Various strategies have been used to solve this problem. Liposomal therapy, a technique whereby the chemotherapy drug is contained within a fat globule (a liposome), which helps it selectively target the cancer cells more effectively, was introduced in the mid-2000's. Doxorubicin has recently been reformulated in this way [Lorusso 2007].

The accumulation of albumin in solid tumors and the high toxicity of standard formulations of drugs such as paclitaxel led to the development of albumin-based drug delivery systems for tumor targeting (reviewed in [Kratz 2008]). An albumin paclitaxel nanoparticle (nab-paclitaxel) was evaluated clinically and is now FDA-approved for treating metastatic breast cancer. Nab-paclitaxel has several practical advantages over standard paclitaxel formulations, including a shorter infusion time and no need for premedications for hypersensitivity reactions.

Another recent development in the field of chemotherapy is the introduction of drug-antibody conjugates, in which monoclonal antibodies can be used to guide the chemotherapy drug to the cancer cells. One of these conjugates is trastuzumab-DM1, where trastuzumab is an anti-HER2/neu antibody and DM1 a microtubule-binding drug. This conjugate has shown activity in metastatic breast carcinoma [Senter 2009].

In 2010, the most used chemotherapy drugs for treating breast cancer patients include:

- the anthracyclines doxorubicin and epirubicin
- he taxanes paclitaxel, docetaxel and ixabepilone [Frye 2010]
- the antimetabolites 5-fluorouracil, capecitabine and gemcitabine
- the alkylating agent cyclophosphamide.

These agents are used alone or in various combinations. Major combinations are:

- doxorubicin-cyclophosphamide
- epirubicin-cyclophosphamide
- fluorouracil–doxorubicin–cyclophosphamide
- fluorouracil-epirubicin-cyclophosphamide
- doxorubicin-taxane
- epirubicin-taxane
- doxorubicin-taxane-cyclophosphamide
- capecitabine-docetaxel
- gemcitabine-paclitaxel
- ixabepilone-capecitabine

In 2010, chemotherapy is generally part of a multimodal treatment employing surgery, chemotherapy, and radiotherapy.

References

Aapro MS. Neoadjuvant therapy in breast cancer: can we define its role? *Oncologist*. 2001;6 (Suppl 3):36-9.

Arcamone F, Franceschi G, Penco S, Selva A. Adriamycin (14-hydroxydaunomycin), a novel antitumor antibiotic. *Tetrahedron Lett*. 1969 Mar;13:1007-10.

Arnold H, Bourseaux F, Brock N: Neuartige Krebs-Chemotherapeutika aus der Gruppe der zyklischen N-Lost-Phosphamidester. *Naturwissenschaften*. 1958;45:64.

Bonadonna G, Brusamolino E, Valagussa P, Rossi A, Brugnatelli L, Brambilla C, De Lena M, Tancini G, Bajetta E, Musumeci R, Veronesi U. Combination chemotherapy as an adjuvant treatment in operable breast cancer. *N. Engl. J. Med*. 1976 Feb 19;294(8):405-10.

Browder T, Butterfield CE, Kräling BM, Shi B, Marshall B, O'Reilly MS, Folkman J. Antiangiogenic scheduling of chemotherapy improves efficacy against experimental drug-resistant cancer. *Cancer Res*. 2000 Apr 1;60(7):1878-86.

Carbone PP. The role of chemotherapy in the treatment of cancer of the breast. *Am. J. Clin. Pathol*. 1975 Dec;64(6):774-9.

DeVita VT Jr, Chu E. A history of cancer chemotherapy. *Cancer Res*. 2008 Nov 1;68(21):8643-53.

Farber S, Diamond LK. Temporary remissions in acute leukemia in children produced by folic acid antagonist, 4-aminopteroyl-glutamic acid. *N. Engl. J.Med.* 1948 Jun 3;238(23):787-93.

Fisher B, Carbone P, Economou SG, Frelick R, Glass A, Lerner H, Redmond C, Zelen M, Band P, Katrych DL, Wolmark N, Fisher ER. 1-Phenylalanine mustard (L-PAM) in the management of primary breast cancer. A report of early findings. *N. Engl. J. Med.* 1975 Jan 16;292(3):117-22.

Frei E 3rd, Karon M, Levin RH, Freireich EJ, Taylor RJ, Hananian J, Selawry O, Holland JF, Hoogstraten B, Wolman IJ, Abir E, Sawitsky A, Lee S, Mills SD, Burgert EO Jr, Spurr CL, Patterson RB, Ebaugh FG, James GW 3rd, Moon JH. The effectiveness of combinations of antileukemic agents in inducing and maintaining remission in children with acute leukemia. *Blood.* 1965 Nov;26(5):642-56.

Frei E 3rd. Curative cancer chemotherapy. *Cancer Res.* 1985 Dec;45(12 Pt 1):6523-37.

Freireich EJ. Min Chiu Li: a perspective in cancer therapy. *Clin. Cancer Res.* 2002 Sep;8(9):2764-5.

Frye DK. Advances in breast cancer treatment: the emerging role of ixabepilone. *Expert Rev. Anticancer Ther.* 2010 Jan;10(1):23-32.

Ganzina F. 4'-epi-doxorubicin, a new analogue of doxorubicin: a preliminary overview of preclinical and clinical data. *Cancer Treat. Rev.* 1983 Mar;10(1):1-22.

Gilman A, Philips FS. The Biological Actions and Therapeutic Applications of the B-Chloroethyl Amines and Sulfides. *Science.* 1946 Apr 5;103(2675):409-36.

Goldie JH. The rationale for the use of preoperative chemotherapy. *Prog. Clin. Biol. Res.* 1985;201:5-14.

Goodman LS, Wintrobe MM, Dameshek W, Goodman MJ, Gilman A, McLennan MT. Landmark article Sept. 21, 1946: Nitrogen mustard therapy. Use of methyl-bis(beta-chloroethyl)amine hydrochloride and tris(beta-chloroethyl)amine hydrochloride for Hodgkin's disease, lymphosarcoma, leukemia and certain allied and miscellaneous disorders. By Louis S. Goodman, Maxwell M. Wintrobe, William Dameshek, Morton J. Goodman, Alfred Gilman and Margaret T. McLennan. JAMA. 1984 May 4;251(17):2255-61.

Heidelberger C, Chaudhuri NK, Danneberg P, Mooren D, Griesbach L, Duschinsky R, Schnitzer RJ, Pleven E, Scheiner J. Fluorinated pyrimidines, a new class of tumour-inhibitory compounds. *Nature*. 1957 Mar 30;179(4561):663-6.

Kratz F. Albumin as a drug carrier: design of prodrugs, drug conjugates and nanoparticles. *J. Control Release*. 2008 Dec 18;132(3):171-83.

Leaf C. Why we're losing the war on cancer (and how to win it). *Fortune*. 2004 Mar 22;149(6):76-82, 84-6, 88 passim.

Li MC, Hertz R, Bergenstal DM. Therapy of choriocarcinoma and related trophoblastic tumors with folic acid and purine antagonists. *N. Engl. J. Med*. 1958 Jul 10;259(2):66-74.

Lorusso V, Manzione L, Silvestris N. Role of liposomal anthracyclines in breast cancer. *Ann. Oncol*. 2007 Jun;18 Suppl 6:vi70-3.

Noer RJ. Adjuvant chemotherapy. Thio-Tepa with radical mastectomy in the treatment ofbreast cancer. *Am. J. Surg*. 1963 Sep;106:405-12.

Papaioannou AN. Preoperative chemotherapy: advantages and clinical application in stage III breast cancer. *Recent Results Cancer Res*. 1985;98:65-90.

Schabel FM Jr. Concepts for systemic treatment of micrometastases. *Cancer*. 1975 Jan;35(1):15-24.

Senter PD. Potent antibody drug conjugates for cancer therapy. *Curr. Opin.Chem. Biol*. 2009 Jun;13(3):235-44.

Singletary SE. Multidisciplinary frontiers in breast cancer management: a surgeon's perspective. *Cancer*. 2007 Mar 15;109(6):1019-29.

Skipper HE, Schabel FM Jr, Wilcox WS. Experimental evaluation of potential anticancer agents. XIII. On the criteria and kinetics associated with "curability" of experimental leukemia. *Cancer Chemother. Rep*. 1964 Feb;35:1-111.

Skipper HE. Historic milestones in cancer biology: a few that are important in cancer treatment (revisited) *Semin. Oncol*. 1979 Dec;6(4):506-14.

Strebhardt K, Ullrich A. Paul Ehrlich's magic bullet concept: 100 years of progress. *Nat. Rev. Cancer*. 2008 Jun;8(6):473-80.

Travis K. Bernard Fisher reflects on a half-century's worth of breast cancer research. *J. Natl. Cancer Inst*. 2005 Nov 16;97(22):1636-7.

Welch HG, Mogielnicki J. Presumed benefit: lessons from the American experience with marrow transplantation for breast cancer. *BMJ*. 2002 May 4;324(7345):1088-92.

Young RC, DeVita VT. Cell cycle characteristics of human solid tumors in vivo. *Cell Tissue Kinet*. 1970 Jul;3(3):285-90.

Chapter 7

Twentieth Century and Beyond Endocrine Therapy of Breast Cancer

Abstract

Hormonodependence of a least some breast tumors was suspected since the end of the 19th century. The mechanisms of breast cancer cell response to estrogens, and their complexity, were progressively unveiled during the 20th century. Major breakthroughs were the identification of estrogen receptors and the introduction of the antiestrogen tamoxifen in clinics. Other antiestrogens have been developed since. Another therapeutical approach, ovarian suppression, already used in the early 1900's, was recently revived with the introduction of goserelin. Another major recent step was the discovery of aromatase inhibitors, able to prevent estrogen production in postmenopausal women. Three of these, exemestane, anastrozole and letrozole are increasingly used.

Observations from the end of 19th century, notably those of Albert Schinzinger and Thomas Beatson (see chapter 3), had suggested the importance of the hormonal milieu on breast cancer and supported the use of oophorectomy. In 1900, *James* Stanley *Newton* Boyd (1856–1916) provided summary data from an analysis of fifty-four cases of oophorectomy in breast cancer, indicating that one third of patients clearly benefited from the operation [Boyd 1900]. The survival period for those patients showing improvement was about 3 times as long as observed for the non-responders. In

1905, Hugh Lett (1876-1964) presented a series of 99 inoperable cases, in which oophorectomy was followed by an improvement in 36, 3% of the cases [Lett 1905]. Depressingly, however, it seemed that even in the cases responding to the operation, the cancer tended to recur within a year in the majority.

The high rate of mortality associated with surgical oophorectomy discouraged many surgeons from performing this operation during the early years of the 20th century. Ovarian ablation by surgery further declined with the arrival of radiotherapy as an alternative means of stopping ovarian function. It was introduced in 1922 by François-*Victor* Foveau de Courmelles (1862-1943) [de Courmelles 1922]. Ovarian irradiation was not routinely used until the mid-20th century, but in turn was brought into disfavor due to the opinion that there were no long-term benefits from these treatments and also due to concerns about the potential long-term toxicities of pelvic irradiation [Prowell and Davidson 2004].

In 1992, a meta-analysis of updated data from clinical trials of adjuvant oophorectomy by radiation and by surgery conducted in the 1960's and 1970's, concluded that, contrary to general opinion at the time, there were long-term benefits from these treatments, with increases in disease-free and overall survival [Early Breast Cancer Trialists' Collaborative Group. 1992].

A detailed overview of the ovarian ablation studies activated before 1990 was published in 1996 [Early Breast Cancer Trialists' Collaborative Group. 1996]. In women aged less than 50 years, ablation of functioning ovaries significantly improved long-term survival, at least in the absence of chemotherapy. In contrast, in women aged 50 or over, when randomized, most of whom would have been postmenopausal, there was only a non-significant improvement.

Ovarian suppression in the management of breast cancer has had resurgence in the 1990's, following the development of luteinizing hormone-releasing hormone (LHRH) analogues: goserelin, triptorelin and leuprolide [Love and Philips 2002]. One of these – goserelin – was licensed for premenopausal and peri-menopausal women with estrogen-dependent early or advanced disease. Various adjuvant trials were carried out and have been reported recently, which show LHRH agonists are as effective as surgical oophorectomy in premenopausal advanced breast cancer. They offer similar outcomes compared with the antiestrogen tamoxifen (see below), but the endocrine combination appears to be more effective than LHRH agonists alone.

In addition to oophorectomy, adrenalectomy [Huggins and Bergenstal 1951] and hypophysectomy [Luft and Olivecrona 1953] were used as hormone-ablative techniques in breast cancer patients. Adrenalectomy was supported by the fact that adrenal glands were found to be the major source of estrogens in postmenopausal or castrated women. Hypophysectomy was based on the postulate that it would eliminate the pituitary hormones or eliminate a "pituitary factor" which could be involved in the growth of breast cancers. In fact, one mechanism to explain the benefit from hypophysectomy is the drop in estrogen levels following removal of the pituitary gland. Although objective remissions were observed in adrenalectomized or hypophysectomized patients, these operations, generating an important morbidity, have now largely been superseded by the development of medical endocrine therapies [Lønning et al. 2003]. Thus, the antiestrogens, notably tamoxifen, have mostly replaced surgical oophorectomy, the aromatase inhibitors (which block peripheral synthesis of estrogens) have replaced adrenalectomy and the luteinizing hormone releasing hormone (LHRH) agonists have replaced hypophysectomy in the management of patients with metastatic breast cancer.

Although oophorectomy was practiced from the end of the 19th century, the mechanism through which this operation could prevent mammary tumors was unknown until 1923, when Edgar Allen (1892-1943) and Edward *Aldebert* Doisy (1893-1986) identified a principle, that they called estrogen (in fact estrone, the principal steroid) in mouse ovarian follicular fluid [Allen and Doisy 1923].

In 1933, Antoine *MarcellinBernard* Lacassagne (1884-1971) first showed that estrogen could induce mammary tumors in mice [Lacassagne 1933; Lacassagne 1936a, 1936b]. He speculated that compounds able to antagonize estrogen action will be discovered.

In 1935, the group of Ernst Laqueur (1880-1947) isolated the androgen testosterone from the testes of a bull [Tausk 1973]. Four years later, Alfred *Alexander* Loeser (1889-1963) and Paul Ulrich and recommended its use in certain forms of breast cancers. Androgenic compounds, notably medroxyprogesterone acetate (MPA), have been used to treat advanced breast cancer, in order to oppose the activity of estrogen. However, their use for this purpose has declined with the advent of tamoxifen [Lundgren 1992].

In 1938, Edward *Charles* Dodds (1899-1973) and colleagues obtained diethylstilboestrol (DES), the first potent synthetic estrogen [Dodds et al. 1938]. DES was subsequently used for the treatment of breast cancer.Unfortunately, DES was also used by millions of pregnant women to prevent miscarriages and many other disorders in pregnancy. In 1971, it became clear that this apparently innocent treatment proved to be a time bomb for the infants exposed to DES during the first trimester of pregnancy. DES is now associated with an increased risk of breast cancer, clear cell adenocarcinoma of the vagina and cervix, and reproductive anomalies (reviewed in [Veurink *et al.* 2005]).

In 1944, Alexander Haddow (1907-1976) and colleagues used high-dose estrogen therapy in breast cancer patients. This first "chemical therapy" caused tumor regressions in postmenopausal patients [Haddow *et al.* 1944]. Before current endocrine therapies were available, advanced postmenopausal breast cancer patients were commonly treated with high dose estrogen. It is still unclear how high dose estrogen therapy works [Santen 2007]. However, Haddow noted that this therapy was more successful as a treatment for breast cancer the farther the woman was from the menopause [Haddow 1950]. Estrogen-withdrawal somehow played a role in sensitizing tumors to the antitumor actions of estrogen. It has recently been suggested that estrogen therapy, abandoned since the introduction of tamoxifen, could be used in tamoxifen-resistant, aromatase inhibitors-resistant women [Munster and Carpenter 2009; Lønning 2009].

In 1958, Leonard Joseph Lerner (b. 1922) discovered ethamoxytriphetol (MER-25), the first non-steroidal antiestrogen [Lerner *et al.* 1958]. MER-25 was investigated in the clinics in a wide range of gynecological conditions, including breast and endometrial cancer. Unfortunately toxic side effects, including unexpected central nervous system symptoms (hallucinations, psychotic episodes, nightmares, disturbed sleep...) precluded further investigation [Lerner and Jordan 1990].

Still in 1958, the progesterone derivative megestrol acetate was synthesized [Petrow and Hartley 1996]. It was first used in (advanced) breast cancer in 1974 [Ansfield *et al.* 1974] and is still the most commonly used progestin in breast cancer patients. Progestins can be fairly effective for the treatment of metastatic breast cancer, although it is not clear how they work. These are effective endocrine therapies and are typically used third line, after failure of selective aromatase inhibitors and tamoxifen. As single-agent therapy, the average overall response rate to megestrol acetate therapy is 30%. Another frequently used progestin is medroxyprogesterone acetate (MPA, see above) [Pasqualini and Ebert 1999].

The existence of an estrogen receptor (ER) was proposed in the early 1960's, notably based on the fact that radioactive estradiol injected to animals bound to and was retained by the estrogen target tissues: the uterus, vagina, and pituitary gland. In contrast, radioactive estradiol bound to, but was not retained, by non-target tissues, e.g. muscle, lung, heart ([Jensen 1962], reviewed in [Jordan 2009]). It was proposed that ER was probably a protein [Noteboom and Gorski 1965]. The first ER was is isolated from rat uterus and characterized in 1966 [Toft and Gorski 1966; Toft *et al.* 1967].

In 1967, the non-steroidal antiestrogen tamoxifen (previously known as ICI 46,474) was introduced [Harper and Walpole 1967]. Initial research had focused on its use as a contraceptive, but it proved unsuccessful for this indication. Other work indicated that it had selective effects on certain types of tissue, including breast tissue. This led to speculation that it might be effective for treating cancer. Studies in the 1970's showed that tamoxifen was a competitive inhibitor of estradiol binding to ER and that it inhibited the binding of estrogen to estrogen target tissues *in vivo*. *In vitro*, in ER-positive breast cancer cells cultures, tamoxifen was shown to inhibit proliferation, an effect reversed by estradiol and not shown in cell lines unresponsive to estradiol [Lerner and Jordan 1990].

During the late 1960's and early 1970's, numerous methods were described to identify and quantitate ER levels in tumor biopsies and these data were subsequently correlated with clinical outcomes in metastatic breast cancer. It was concluded that breast tumors devoid of ER were unlikely to respond to endocrine ablation and therefore should not be treated with this modality (reviewed in [McGuire *et al.* 1975]).The breast cancer chemoprevention concept appeared in 1976. According to it, the development of epithelial cancer, including breast cancer, is a disease process that takes many years to reach its final, invasive stage in humans, and this disease process has the potential to be controlled by physiological or pharmacological means during its preneoplastic stages [Sporn 1976].Still in 1976, *Virgil* Craig Jordan (b. 1947) and colleagues showed that tamoxifen could prevent mammary carcinogenesis in DMBA-treated rats (see chapter 12) [Jordan 1976]. In the following decades, studies demonstrated its ability to reduce breast cancer incidence in women. However, concerns about the potential of tamoxifen to increase the risk of endometrial cancer and the carcinogenic potential of the drug as a hepatocarcinogen (reviewed in [Jordan 2009]) favored the recourse to raloxifene (see below) for breast cancer chemoprevention. In 1977, tamoxifen was FDA-approved for treatment of metastatic breast cancer.While tamoxifen was initially given to patients for a short period (1 year), its use was extended up to 5 years, with substantial improvement of survival of women with ER-positive tumors [Early Breast Cancer Trialists' Collaborative Group 1998, Early Breast Cancer Trialists' Collaborative Group 2005]. Tamoxifen is a "selective estrogen receptor modifier", or SERM. SERMs directly bind to the ER and block its transcriptional activity. Estrogen is produced principally by the ovaries in premenopausal women. After the menopause, production of estrogen from the ovaries stops but the adrenal glands secrete androgens that can be converted by aromatase to estrogens in tissues such as fat and in breast cancer cells. Attempts to block adrenal function as a treatment for breast cancer led to the serendipitous finding, in the late 1970's-early 1980's, that a non-steroidal P450 steroidogenesis inhibitor, aminoglutethimide, served as a potent but non-selective aromatase inhibitor (reviewed in [Santen *et al.* 2009]). In 1982, Angela *Hartley* Brodie (b. 1934) discovered that formestane (4-hydroxyandrostenedione), a selective aromatase inhibitor, could stop the growth of breast cancer in women whose tumors were resistant to tamoxifen. Brodie hypothesized that the aromatase inhibitors could prove to be a more effective alternative to tamoxifen [Brodie 1982]. Formestane was introduced on the market in 1994. It was the first new treatment for breast cancer in a decade. After many refinements, three aromatase inhibitors were approved and are currently used for treating advanced breast cancer in postmenopausal women: exemestane, anastrozole and letrozole. Subsequent clinical trials have shown that anastrozole and letrozole are more effective than tamoxifen for advanced breast cancer and as adjuvant therapy in early disease. They are also effective after tamoxifen in some patients. These drugs have become the new gold standard of endocrine therapy. In 1983, raloxifene, originally known as keoxifene, LY139481 or LY156758, was introduced [Clemens *et al.* 1983; Wakeling and Valcaccia 1983]. Like tamoxifen, raloxifen is a SERM. Initially used as a nonsteroidal antiestrogen for the treatment of breast cancer, the drug failed in that indication and further development was abandoned. However, several years later, raloxifene was shown to maintain bone density in osteoporotic or osteopenic women [Ettinger *et al.* 1999], and simultaneously reduce the incidence of invasive breast cancer without causing an increase in the incidence of endometrial cancer [Cummings *et al.* 1999]. Raloxifene went on to be tested against tamoxifen in the Study of Tamoxifen and Raloxifene trial [Vogel *et al.* 2006] and was FDA approved both for the treatment and prevention of osteoporosis in postmenopausal women and for the reduction of invasive breast cancer incidence in postmenopausal women at elevated risk (reviewed in [Jordan 2009]).In 1986, a first human ER was cloned. It was later renamed ER–alpha (ERα) [Greene *et al.* 1986; Green *et al.* 1986]. In 1991-1992, fulvestrant (previously known as ICI 182,780), an antiestrogen with clinical potential was introduced [Wakeling and Bowler 1992]. Fulvestrant was the first "selective estrogen receptor down-regulators", or SERD, used in clinical trials. SERDs bind to estrogen receptor and induce its degradation. Fulvestrant is also called a pure antiestrogen or estrogen antagonist. It is increasingly used in breast cancer patients, notably following disease progression or recurrence on tamoxifen and/or aromatase inhibitors. For a review on fulvestrant, see [Buzdar 2008]. In 1995, the first coregulator of ER action, termed steroid receptor coactivator-1 (SRC-1), was discovered [Oñate*et al.* 1995]. Various ER coactivators and corepressors have been identified since. Evidence has accumulated that the broad spectrum of ligands that bind to the ER can create a broad range of ER complexes that are either fully estrogenic or antiestrogenic at a particular target site. Thus, a mechanistic model of estrogen action and antiestrogen action has emerged based on the shape of the ligand that programs the complex to adopt a particular shape that ultimately interacts with coactivators or corepressors in target cells to determine the estrogenic or antiestrogenic response, respectively [Jordan 2009].In 1996, a second human ER, estrogen receptor-beta (β), was discovered [Kuiper *et al.* 1996]. The ER proteins encode on different chromosomes and have homology as members of the steroid receptor superfamily, but there are distinct patterns of distribution and distinct and subtle differences in structure and ligand binding affinity. An additional dimension that may be significant for tissue modulation is the ratio of ERα and ERβ at a target site. A high ERα/ERβ ratio correlates well with very high levels of cellular proliferation, whereas the predominance of functional ERβ over ERα correlates with low levels of proliferation [Jordan 2009]. Subtype-specific ligands have been developed. Several studies suggest that the majority of ER-positive tumors contain both subtypes, but that some tumors contain only ERβ and may have distinct clinical behaviors and responses. Expression of ERβ together with ERα favors positive responses to endocrine therapy in most studies, and additional studies to determine if the addition of ERβ to ERα as a tumor marker is of clinical benefit are warranted. In contrast, the positive association between ERβ and HER2 expression in high-grade ERα-negative breast cancer does not favor positive responses to endocrine therapy (see notably [Fox *et al.* 2008]).

References

Allen E, Doisy EA. An ovarian hormone. Preliminary report on its localization, extraction and partial purification, and action in test animals. *JAMA*. 1923;81:810-21.

Ansfield FJ, Davis HL Jr, Ellerby RA, Ramirez G. A clinical trial of megestrol acetate in advanced breast cancer. *Cancer*. 1974 Apr;33(4):907-10.

Boyd S. On oophorectomy in cancer of the breast. *BMJ* 1900;2:1161–7.

Brodie AM. Overview of recent development of aromatase inhibitors. *Cancer Res*. 1982 Aug;42(8 Suppl):3312s-3314s.

Buzdar AU. Fulvestrant--a novel estrogen receptor antagonist for the treatment of advanced breast cancer. *Drugs Today* (Barc). 2008 Sep;44(9):679-92.

Clemens JA, Bennett DR, Black LJ, Jones CD. Effects of a new antiestrogen, keoxifene (LY156758), on growth of carcinogen-induced mammary tumors and on LH and prolactin levels. *Life Sci*. 1983 Jun 20;32(25):2869-75.

Cummings SR, Eckert S, Krueger KA, Grady D, Powles TJ, Cauley JA, Norton L, Nickelsen T, Bjarnason NH, Morrow M, Lippman ME, Black D, Glusman JE, Costa A, Jordan VC. The effect of raloxifene on risk of breast cancer in postmenopausal women: results from the MORE randomized trial. Multiple Outcomes of Raloxifene Evaluation. *JAMA*. 1999 Jun 16;281(23):2189-97.

de Courmelles FV. La radiotherapie indirecte ou dirigée par les correlation organique. *Arch. Elect. Med* 1922;32:264.

Dodds EC, Lawson W, Noble RL. Biological effects of the synthetic oestrogenic substance 4:4'-dihydroxy-alpha:beta-diethylstilbene. *Lancet* 1938;1:1389–91.

Early Breast Cancer Trialists' Collaborative Group. Tamoxifen for early breast cancer: an overview of the randomised trials. *Lancet*. 1998 May 16;351(9114):1451-67.

Early Breast Cancer Trialists' Collaborative Group (EBCTCG). Effects of chemotherapy and hormonal therapy for early breast cancer on recurrence and 15-year survival: an overview of the randomised trials. *Lancet*. 2005 May 14-20;365(9472):1687-717.

Ettinger B, Black DM, Mitlak BH, Knickerbocker RK, Nickelsen T, Genant HK, Christiansen C, Delmas PD, Zanchetta JR, Stakkestad J, Glüer CC, Krueger K, Cohen FJ, Eckert S, Ensrud KE, Avioli LV, Lips P, Cummings SR. Reduction of vertebral fracture risk in postmenopausal women with osteoporosis treated with raloxifene: results from a 3-year randomized clinical trial. Multiple Outcomes of Raloxifene Evaluation (MORE) Investigators. *JAMA*. 1999 Aug 18;282(7):637-45.

Fox EM, Davis RJ, Shupnik MA. ERbeta in breast cancer--onlooker, passive player, or active protector? *Steroids*. 2008 Oct;73(11):1039-51.

Green S, Walter P, Kumar V, Krust A, Bornert JM, Argos P, Chambon P. Human oestrogen receptor cDNA: sequence, expression and homology to v-erb-A. *Nature*. 1986 Mar 13-19;320(6058):134-9.

Greene GL, Gilna P, Waterfield M, Baker A, Hort Y, Shine J. Sequence and expression of human estrogen receptor complementary DNA. *Science*. 1986 Mar 7;231(4742):1150-4.

Haddow A, Watkinson JM, Paterson E. Influence of synthetic oestrogens upon advanced malignant disease. *Br. Med. J*. 1944;2:393–8.

Haddow A. The chemotherapy of cancer. *Br. Med. J*. 1950 Dec 2;2(4691):1271-2.

Harper MJ, Walpole AL. A new derivative of triphenylethylene: effect on implantation and mode of action in rats. *J. Reprod Fertil*. 1967 Feb;13(1):101-19.

Huggins C, Bergenstal DM. Surgery of the adrenals. *J. Am. Med. Assoc*. 1951 Sep 8;147(2):101-6.

Jensen EV. On the mechanism of estrogen action. *Perspect Biol. Med*. 1962;6:47-59.

Jordan VC. Effect of tamoxifen (ICI 46,474) on initiation and growth of DMBA-induced rat mammary carcinomata. *Eur. J. Cancer*. 1976 Jun;12(6):419-24.

Jordan VC. A century of deciphering the control mechanisms of sex steroid action in breast and prostate cancer: the origins of targeted therapy and chemoprevention. *Cancer Res*. 2009 Feb 15;69(4):1243-54.

Kuiper GG, Enmark E, Pelto-Huikko M, Nilsson S, Gustafsson JA. Cloning of a novel receptor expressed in rat prostate and ovary. *Proc. Natl. Acad. Sci. U S A*. 1996 Jun 11;93(12):5925-30.

Lacassagne A. Influence d'un facteur familial dans la production par la folliculine, de cancers mammaires chez la souris male. *J. Soc. Biol*.1933;114:427–9.

Lacassagne A. A comparative study of the carcinogenic action of certain oestrogenic hormones. *Am. J. Cancer* 1936a;28:735–40.

Lacassagne A. Hormonal pathogenesis of adenocarcinoma of the breast. *Am. J. Cancer* 1936b;27:217–25.

Lerner LJ, Holthaus FJ Jr, Thompson CR. A non-steroidal estrogen antiagonist 1-(p-2-diethylaminoethoxyphenyl)-1-phenyl-2-p-methoxyphenyl ethanol. *Endocrinology*. 1958 Sep;63(3):295-318.

Lerner LJ, Jordan VC. Development of antiestrogens and their use in breast cancer: eighth Cain memorial award lecture. *Cancer Res*. 1990 Jul 15;50(14):4177-89.

Lett, H. An analysis of ninety-nine cases of inoperable carcinoma of the breast treated by oophorectomy, *Lancet* 1905 Jan 28;1:227-8.

Lønning PE, Geisler J, Bhatnager A. Development of aromatase inhibitors and their pharmacologic profile. *Am. J. Clin. Oncol.* 2003 Aug;26(4):S3-8.

Lønning PE. Additive endocrine therapy for advanced breast cancer - back to the future. *Acta Oncol.* 2009;48(8):1092-101.

Love RR, Philips J. Oophorectomy for breast cancer: history revisited. *J.Natl. Cancer Inst.* 2002 Oct 2;94(19):1433-4.

Luft R, Olivecrona H. Experiences with hypophysectomy in man. *J.Neurosurg.* 1953 May;10(3):301-16.

Lundgren S. Progestins in breast cancer treatment. *A. review. Acta Oncol.* 1992;31(7):709-22.

McGuire WL, Chamness GC, Costlow ME, Richert NJ. Steroids and human breast cancer. *J. Steroid. Biochem.* 1975 May;6(5):723-7.

Munster PN, Carpenter JT. Estradiol in breast cancer treatment: reviving the past. *JAMA.* 2009 Aug 19;302(7):797-8.

Noteboom WD, Gorski J. Stereospecific binding of estrogens in the rat uterus. *Arch. Biochem. Biophys.* 1965 Sep;111(3):559-68.

Oñate SA, Tsai SY, Tsai MJ, O'Malley BW. Sequence and characterization of a coactivator for the steroid hormone receptor superfamily. *Science.* 1995 Nov 24;270(5240):1354-7.

Pasqualini JR, Ebert C. Biological effects of progestins in breast cancer. *Gynecol. Endocrinol.* 1999 Jun;13 Suppl 4:11-9.

Petrow V, Hartley F. The rise and fall of the British Drug Houses, Ltd. *Steroids.* 1996 Aug;61(8):476-82.

Prowell TM, Davidson NE. What is the role of ovarian ablation in the management of primary and metastatic breast cancer today? *Oncologist.* 2004;9(5):507-17.

Santen RJ. The oestrogen paradox: a hypothesis. *Endokrynol. Pol.* 2007 May-Jun;58(3):222-7.

Santen RJ, Brodie H, Simpson ER, Siiteri PK, Brodie A. History of aromatase: saga of an important biological mediator and therapeutic target. *Endocr. Rev.* 2009 Jun;30(4):343-75.

Sporn MB. Approaches to prevention of epithelial cancer during the preneoplastic period. *Cancer Res.* 1976 Jul;36(7 PT 2):2699-702.

Tausk M. The 1973 Ernst Laqueur Memorial Lecture. Arma virosque. *Acta Endocrinol* (Copenh). 1973 Nov;74(3):417-33.

Toft D, Gorski J. A receptor molecule for estrogens: isolation from the rat uterus and preliminary characterization. *Proc. Natl. Acad. Sci. U S A.* 1966 Jun;55(6):1574-81.

Toft D, Shyamala G, Gorski J. A receptor molecule for estrogens: studies using a cell-free system. Proc Natl Acad Sci U S A. 1967 Jun;57(6):1740-3.

Veurink M, Koster M, Berg LT. The history of DES, lessons to be learned. *Pharm. World Sci.* 2005 Jun;27(3):139-43.

Vogel VG, Costantino JP, Wickerham DL, Cronin WM, Cecchini RS, Atkins JN, Bevers TB, Fehrenbacher L, Pajon ER Jr, Wade JL 3rd, Robidoux A, Margolese RG, James J, Lippman SM, Runowicz CD, Ganz PA, Reis SE, McCaskill-Stevens W, Ford LG, Jordan VC, Wolmark N; National Surgical Adjuvant Breast and Bowel Project (NSABP). Effects of tamoxifen vs raloxifene on the risk of developing invasive breast cancer and other disease outcomes: the NSABP Study of Tamoxifen and Raloxifene (STAR) P-2 trial. JAMA. 2006 Jun 21;295(23):2727-41.

Wakeling AE, Valcaccia B. Antioestrogenic and antitumour activities of a series of non-steroidal antioestrogens. *J. Endocrinol.* 1983 Dec;99(3):455-64.

Wakeling AE, Bowler J. ICI 182,780, a new antioestrogen with clinical potential. *J. Steroid Biochem. Mol. Biol.* 1992 Sep;43(1-3):173-7.

Chapter 8

Twentieth Century and Beyond Targeted Therapy of Breast Cancer (Including Immunotherapy)

Abstract

Despite surgery, radiotherapy, chemotherapy and endocrine therapy, metastatic breast cancers are still incurable. With the hope to overcome this resistance, new agents are in development. They are directed against specific targets, of which the expression and sensitivity may vary among breast cancer patients. They should be less toxic for the patients. On the other hand, they may require a careful selection of patients who would benefit from them. While trastuzumab, lapatinib and bevacizumab have been recently approved by the FDA, a number of other compounds, representing various families and approaches, have entered clinical trials during the last ten years. Targeted therapy is still in its infancy.

While a series of biological anticancer drugs were intensively studied in various laboratories during the 1990's, it was not before 1997 that the first biotechnology product, a monoclonal antibody called rituximab [Anderson *et al.* 1997], was approved by the FDA to treat patients with cancer. Rituximab is directed against the B-cell-specific antigen CD20. It is used to treat non-Hodgkin's lymphoma (NHL), but not breast cancer.

Trastuzumab, the first molecular based targeted treatment for breast cancer, was FDA-approved in 1998. Trastuzumab is a monoclonal antibody against HER2/neu. Monoclonal antibodies are derived from the hybridoma technology initially developed by Georges *Jean Franz* Köhler (1946–1995) and César Milstein (1927–2002) in the 1970's. These investigators demonstrated that antibody-producing cells of virtually any desired specificity could be fused with a myeloma cell line, the result being unlimited amounts of homogeneous (monoclonal) antibodies carrying that specificity [Köhler and Milstein 1975]. HER2/neu is a receptor tyrosine kinase involved in cell growth and differentiation. In around 20–30 per cent of breast cancers the HER2/neu protein is over-expressed, resulting mainly from the amplification of the corresponding *ERBB2* gene, and this causes an aggressive form of the disease [Varley *et al.* 1987; Lacroix *et al.* 2004; Ross *et al.* 2009]. Trastuzumab binds to the domain IV of the extracellular segment of HER2/neu. Breast cancer cells treated with trastuzumab undergo arrest during the G1 phase of the cell cycle. For a review on trastuzumab and anti-HER2/neu therapies in breast cancer, see [Daniele and Sapino 2009]).

Trastuzumab is indicated by the US Food and Drug Administration (FDA):as adjuvant in the treatment of HER2/neu overexpressing node positive or node negative (ER/PR negative or with one high risk feature) breast cancer:

1) as part of a treatment regimen consisting of doxorubicin, cyclophosphamide, and either paclitaxel or docetaxel;
2) with docetaxel and carboplatin;
3) as a single agent following multi-modality anthracycline based therapy;

In the treatment of metastatic breast cancer:

1) in combination with paclitaxel for first-line treatment of HER2-overexpressing metastatic breast cancer;
2) as a single agent for treatment of HER2-overexpressing breast cancer in patients who have received one or more chemotherapy regimens formetastatic disease.

Currently, multiple trials are testing combinations of trastuzumab and other drugs. Adverse effects associated with trastuzumab use are cardiotoxicity and a higher rate of development of cerebral metastases. Moreover, although trastuzumab has produced dramatic results for many women with breast cancer, a significant proportion of these eventually become resistant to the drug [Nanda 2007]. It is the reason why drugs such as lapatinib (see below) were developed.

In 2003 were reported the first clinical studies of bevacizumab in breast cancer patients [Cobleigh *et al.* 2003]. Bevacizumab is the first biological drug directed against angiogenesis. Angiogenesis is the formation of new blood vessels. It is necessary for the growth and development of normal tissues and for wound healing. Once tumors reach a certain size they also rely on new blood vessels for further growth and to spread to other sites. Thus, angiogenesis is an important mediator of growth and metastasis in most cancers. Angiogenesis inhibitors stop angiogenesis by preventing angiogenic factors from binding to tumor cells. Bevacizumab is a monoclonal antibody that binds to vascular endothelial growth factor-A (VEGF-A) and reduces the availability of this latter for its receptors (VEGFR)-1 and VEGFR-2. It thereby prevents endothelial cell survival, proliferation, permeability, migration, and invasion [Yang 2009].

In 2004 were reported the first clinical studies of lapatinib (also known as GW572016) in breast cancer patients. Lapatinib is a dual inhibitor of HER2/neu and epidermal growth factor receptor (EGFR). Dual inhibition of both tyrosine kinases had been found to exert greater biologic effects in the inhibition of signaling pathways promoting breast cancer cell proliferation and survival than inhibition of either receptor alone (reviewed in [Burris 2004] and in [Ross *et al.* 2009]).

In 2007, lapatinib was approved by the FDA for breast cancer patients. It is currently indicated in combination with capecitabine in the treatment of patients with advanced or metastatic breast cancer whose tumors overexpress HER2 and who have received prior therapy including an anthracycline, a taxane, and trastuzumab.

In 2008, bevacizumab was approved by the FDA for breast cancer patients. It is currently indicated in combination with paclitaxel in the treatment of patients who have not received chemotherapy for metastatic HER2 negative breast cancer. The effectiveness of bevacizumab in metastatic breast cancer is based on an improvement in progression free survival. Bevacizumab is not indicated for patients with breast cancer that has progressed following anthracycline and taxane chemotherapy administered for metastatic disease.

Other promising targeted compounds are currently in clinical trials in breast cancer patients. They are listed in Table 2. More details on the various families of compounds are also given.

Table 2. Breast cancer drugs in clinical trials in 2009/2010. Based on the book: "Molecular Therapy of Breast Cancer: Classicism meets Modernity", by Marc Lacroix (Nova Science Publishers, 2009)

Family of compounds	Compounds in clinical trials in breast cancer patients in 2009-2010
HER Family Inhibitors	Trastuzumab; lapatinib; erlotinib; pertuzumab; cetuximab, ertumaxomab; neratinib; trastuzumab-MCC-DM1; BIBW 2992; ARRY-334543
Angiogenesis inhibitors	Bevacizumab; sunitinib; vandetanib; pazopanib; ramucirumab; ABT-869; AV-951; PTC299; AMG 386; aflibercept
IGF-1R inhibitors	Cixutumumab; figitumumab; OSI-906; AMG 479 ;BMS-754807; MK0646; AVE1642
Ras-Raf-MEK-ERK pathway inhibitors	Lonafarnib; tipifarnib; sorafenib; AZD6244
Proteasome inhibitor	Bortezomib
Histone deacetylases inhibitors	Vorinostat; panobinostat; entinostat; belinostat; valproic acid
Mitotic inhibitors (non microtubule-binding)	MLN8237; ispinesib; PD 0332991; UCN-01; SCH 727965
Inhibitors of heat-shock proteins 90 and 27	CNF2024; NVP-AUY922; retaspimycin; OGX-427
Inhibitors of the PI3K/Akt/mTOR pathway	Everolimus; temsirolimus; sirolimus; deferolimus; BGT226; NVP-BEZ235; GSK1059615
Cyclooxygenase-2 inhibitors	Celecoxib; apricoxib
PARP inhibitors	Olaparib; BSI-201; AG014699; ABT-888
Tumor-induced osteolysis inhibitors	Zoledronic acid; ibandronate; risedronate; clodronate; alendronate; denosumab; odanacatib

Family of compounds	Compounds in clinical trials in breast cancer patients in 2009-2010
Vaccines and immunomodulators	Allogeneic GM-CSF-secreting breast cancer vaccine; TTK peptide (mixed with adjuvant Montanide ISA-51; hTERT/Survivin Multi-Peptide Vaccine; AE37 peptide/GM-CSF vaccine; GP2 peptide/GM-CSF vaccine; falimarev; inalimarev; HER2/neu (extracellular domain) peptide vaccine; sialyl Lewis^a-keyhole limpet hemocyanin (KLH) conjugate vaccine; telomerase: 540-548 peptide vaccine; Ad-sig-hMUC-1/ecdCD40L vaccine; AVX701; recombinant fowlpox-CEA(6D)/TRICOM vaccine; recombinant vaccinia-CEA(6D)-TRICOM vaccine; ovarian cancer peptide mix immunotherapeutic vaccine; modified vaccinia Ankara (Bavarian Nordic)-HER2 vaccine; autologous dendritic cell-adenovirus p53 vaccine;pNGVL3-hICD vaccine; mammaglobin-A DNA vaccine; CHP-HER2; CHP-NY-ESO-1; AS1402; CDX-1307; IMP321
Varia	AFP464; aldesleukin; ALT-801; ATN-224; AZD0530; bavituximab; bosutinib; BZL101; CR011-vcMMAE; dasatinib; denileukin diftitox; enzastaurin; GRN163L; imatinib; interleukin-12; lonaprisan; MK-0752; rexin-G; tesmilifene; trabectedin; WX-671

The Families of Compounds: Details

HER Family Inhibitors and Angiogenesis Inhibitors

See above

IGF-1R inhibitors

The insulin-like growth factor-I receptor (IGF-IR) is overexpressed in many types of malignancies, and has been implicated as a principal cause of heightened proliferative and survival signaling. IGF-IR has also been shown to confer resistance to cytotoxic, hormonal, and targeted therapies, suggesting that therapeutics targeting IGF-IR may be effective against a broad range of malignancies. Inhibition of IGF-IR in a variety of tumor types, by a variety of strategies *in vitro* and *in vivo*, has antiproliferative effects and synergizes with other anticancer therapies.

Ras-Raf-MEK-ERK Pathway Inhibitors

Growth factors and mitogens use the Ras-Raf-MEK-ERK signaling cascade to transmit signals from their receptors to regulate gene expression and prevent apoptosis.The members of this pathway provide new opportunities for the development of targeted anti-cancer drugs.

Proteasome Inhibitor

Aberrations in the ubiquitin-proteasome system have been recently connected to the pathogenesis of cancer, so that proteasome is now considered an important target for drug discovery. Small molecules able to inhibit and modulate ubiquitin-proteasome system are a new approach in anti-cancer therapy, supported by pharmacologic, preclinical, and clinical data. Furthermore, several studies have demonstrated that proteasome inhibitors may potentiate the activity of other anti-cancer treatment, in part by down-regulating chemoresistance pathways.

Histone Deacetylases Inhibitors

Histone deacetylases (HDACs) deacetylate the amino-terminal tails of histones, thereby affecting transcription and other nuclear events. HDACs activity is frequently altered in tumors. Many HDAC inhibitors have entered pre-clinical or clinical research as anti-cancer agents and shown satisfying effects.

Mitotic Inhibitors (Non Microtubule-Binding)

Microtubule-binding drugs are mitotic inhibitors associated with significant toxicity. This led to the development of new inhibitors targeting non-microtubule structures involved in cell cycle regulation (cyclin-dependent kinases, checkpoint kinases, Aurora and Polo kinases, microtubule motor proteins).

Inhibitors of Heat-Shock Proteins 90 and 27

The heat-shock protein 90 (Hsp90) multichaperone complex has wide-ranging functions that result from the ability of this sophisticated machinery to assist in the folding and function of a variety of 'client proteins'. Multiple proteins involved in cell-specific oncogenic processes, including steroid hormone receptors and HER2/neu in breast cancer, have been shown to be tightly regulated by the binding of the Hsp90 machinery. This may be seen as a biochemical buffer for the numerous cancer-specific lesions that are characteristic of diverse tumors. Several small-molecule inhibitors of Hsp90 have shown potent antitumor activity in a wide-range of malignancies.

Inhibitors of the PI3K/Akt/Mtor Pathway

The phosphatidylinositol-3-kinase (PI3K)/Akt/mammalian target of rapamycin (mTOR) pathway plays a central role in cell survival and proliferation. Deregulation of this pathway has been implicated in the promotion of cancer cell growth and survival. Inhibition of several steps of this pathway has been shown to confer favorable antitumor activity in a variety of cancer types.

Cyclooxygenase-2 Inhibitors

Cyclooxygenase-2 (COX-2) is an inducible enzyme that catalyzes the rate-limiting step in the production of prostaglandins. It is frequently overexpressed in breast cancer. Specific COX-2 inhibitors have been designed.

PARP Inhibitors

Poly(ADP-ribose) polymerases (PARPs) are defined as a family of cell signaling enzymes present in eukaryotes, which are involved in poly(ADP-ribosylation) of DNA-binding proteins. The best studied of these enzymes

(PARP-1) is involved in the cellular response to DNA damage. Inhibitors of PARP-1 activity in combination with DNA-binding antitumor drugs may constitute a suitable strategy in cancer chemotherapy.

Tumor-Induced Osteolysis Inhibitors

Breast cancer cells may adversely influence bone and mineral metabolism through a broad spectrum of mechanisms including systemic humoral mechanisms and by direct metastatic invasion of bone, which results in bone loss, hypercalcaemia and excruciating bone pain. Molecular inhibitors of tumor-induced osteolysis have been developed, including the bisphosphonates.

Vaccines and Immunomodulators

Vaccines may be prophylactic or therapeutic. Prophylactic vaccines may be useful for diseases in which there is a known etiologic agent. They consist in immunogens introduced into the body before actual disease exposure [Mittendorf et al. 2007]. This approach has been successful in preventing human papillomavirus (HPV)-associated cervical cancer (for a review, see [Dunne et al. 2008]). For most cancers, including breast cancer, no specific infectious agents seem to play a significant causal role. As a consequence, most experimental cancer vaccines to date have been designed to stimulate a cellular immune response against antigens from established tumors and, thus, to be "therapeutic". Trials evaluating these vaccines have administrated them as a therapeutic agent, most often in patients with significant tumor burden [Mittendorf et al. 2007].

Attempts to develop breast tumor vaccines have been done since the late 1990's but have met with limited success. Explanations for this low success rate are multiple: difficulty of identifying specific tumor antigens; low expression level of these specific antigens, which may also be located in a cryptic site or otherwise shielded from surveillance; mild immunogenicity of the antigens, most of which are self-antigens; advanced stage of the patients recruited for vaccine trials; large tumor size, resulting in the fact that cells on the interior of the tumor may not be accessible; release of immunosuppressive factors by tumor cells…

However, due to recent progress in the understanding of the molecular and cellular basis of immunity, immunotherapy is poised to become a major modality of cancer care. A number of distinct cancer vaccine platforms are currently tested in clinical trials. They may be based on molecular biology, targeting distinct antigens that are delivered as peptide, protein, or as genetically engineered plasmid DNA vectors, viruses, or bacteria. Alternatively, they may be based on cell biology, utilizing patient-derived dendritic cells, autologous tumor cells or tumor cell lysates, or allogeneic tumor cells [Interested readers are invited to consult a series of recent publications ([Mittendorf *et al.* 2007, Singletary 2007, Emens 2008, Anderson 2009]).

References

Anderson DR, Grillo-López A, Varns C, Chambers KS, Hanna N. Targeted anti-cancer therapy using rituximab, a chimaeric anti-CD20 antibody (IDEC-C2B8) in the treatment of non-Hodgkin's B-cell lymphoma. *Biochem. Soc. Trans.* 1997 May;25(2):705-8.

Anderson KS. Tumor vaccines for breast cancer. *Cancer Invest.* 2009 May;27(4):361-8.

Burris HA 3rd. Dual kinase inhibition in the treatment of breast cancer: initial experience with the EGFR/ErbB-2 inhibitor lapatinib. *Oncologist.* 2004;9 Suppl 3:10-5.

Cobleigh MA, Langmuir VK, Sledge GW, Miller KD, Haney L, Novotny WF, Reimann JD, Vassel A. A phase I/II dose-escalation trial of bevacizumab in previously treated metastatic breast cancer. *Semin. Oncol.* 2003 Oct;30(5 Suppl 16):117-24.

Daniele L, Sapino A. Anti-HER2 treatment and breast cancer: state of the art, recent patents, and new strategies. *Recent Pat. Anticancer Drug Discov.* 2009 Jan;4(1):9-18.

Dunne EF, Datta SD, E Markowitz L. A review of prophylactic human papillomavirus vaccines: recommendations and monitoring in the US. *Cancer.* 2008 Nov 15;113(10 Suppl):2995-3003.

Emens LA. Cancer vaccines: on the threshold of success. *Expert Opin Emerg Drugs.* 2008 Jun;13(2):295-308.

Köhler G, Milstein C. Continuous cultures of fused cells secreting antibody of predefined specificity. *Nature.* 1975 Aug 7;256(5517):495-7.

Lacroix M, Toillon RA, Leclercq G. Stable 'portrait' of breast tumors during progression: data from biology, pathology and genetics. *Endocr Relat Cancer*. 2004 Sep;11(3):497-522.

Mittendorf EA, Peoples GE, Singletary SE. Breast cancer vaccines: promise for the future or pipe dream? *Cancer*. 2007 Oct 15;110(8):1677-86.

Nanda R. Targeting the human epidermal growth factor receptor 2 (HER2) in the treatment of breast cancer: recent advances and future directions. Rev *RecentClin Trials*. 2007 May;2(2):111-6.

Ross JS, Slodkowska EA, Symmans WF, Pusztai L, Ravdin PM, Hortobagyi GN. The HER-2 receptor and breast cancer: ten years of targeted anti-HER-2 therapy and personalized medicine. *Oncologist*. 2009 Apr;14(4):320-68.

Singletary SE. Multidisciplinary frontiers in breast cancer management: a surgeon's perspective. *Cancer*. 2007 Mar 15;109(6):1019-29.

Varley JM, Swallow JE, Brammar WJ, Whittaker JL, Walker RA. Alterations to either c-erbB-2(neu) or c-myc proto-oncogenes in breast carcinomas correlate with poor short-term prognosis. *Oncogene*. 1987;1(4):423-30.

Yang SX. Bevacizumab and breast cancer: current therapeutic progress and future perspectives. *Expert Rev Anticancer Ther*. 2009 Dec;9(12):1715-25.

Chapter 9

Twentieth Century and Beyond Breast Cancer Staging and Grading

Abstract

By the first half of the 20th century, clinicians became aware that not all breast cancers shared the same prognosis or required the same treatment, and attempts were made to define characteristics that could reliably distinguish those tumors that required aggressive treatment from those that did not.

The various tumor staging systems developed during the century culminated in the "TNM" classification, based on the extent of the primary tumor (T), the absence, presence and extent of regional lymph node involvement (N) and the absence or presence of distant metastases.

Tumor grading systems, aiming to associate histological grades and prognosis, culminated in the "Nottingham modification of the Bloom-Richardson system", which includes three scored morphologic features: degree of tumor tubule formation, tumor mitotic activity, and nuclear grade of tumor cells.

Staging

In 1905, Karl (or Carl) Steinthal (1859-1938) divided breast cancer into three stages according to the size and spread of their tumors [Steinthal 1905]:

- *Stage 1*: Tumors apparently limited to the breast, with no signs of axillary lymph nodes involvement.
- *Stage 2:*Larger tumors adherent to the skin and with palpable axillary lymph nodes.
- *Stage 3*: Tumors adherent to the skin and underlying muscle and having invaded the tissues surrounding the breast and even more distant organs such as bone and liver.

Steinthal decided to stop operating on women with stage III cancer, because he believed this group could not be cured. Staging became popular in Germany and Scandinavia, but did not catch on elsewhere until the 1950s.

Robert *Battey* Greenough (1871-1937), partly drawing on earlier work by the German pathologist David *Paul* von Hansemann (1858-1920) [von Hansemann 1890], who recognized that the morphologic appearance of tumors was associated with the degree of malignancy, proposed in 1925 that breast cancer is more than one disease. He published survival data according to three classes of malignancy, based on microscopic examination of breast cancer specimens: cancers of low malignancy (class I), which were usually cured, those of high malignancy (class III), which were usually lethal, and those of medium malignancy (class II) [Greenough 1925]. In Greenough's group of 73 breast cancer patients, 13/19 (68%), 11/33 (33%) and 0/21 (0%) patients from class I, II, and III, respectively, were still alive after five years, supporting that the treatment of all breast cancers by an uniformly radical method was illogical.

In 1940, James *Ralston Kennedy* Paterson (1897-1981) began to develop the Manchester system, or Manchester classification, a refined clinical staging system for breast cancer. It was a modification of the Steinthal staging system including four stages:

- *Stage 1*: The primary tumor is confined to the breast, is movable, with the only skin attachment being at the tumor site.
- *Stage 2:* Similar tumor features, but there are palpable mobile lymph nodes in the axilla of the same side.
- *Stage 3:* The primary growth is more extensive, involving a wider skin area with muscle fixation, but tumor and lymph nodes are not fixed to the chest wall.

- *Stage 4*: Extension beyond the breast as shown by chest wall fixation of the tumor and axillary nodes, supraclavicular node involvement, and distant metastases.

For years, this staging system was the most common classification referred to in the British and European literature. However, by 1960, there had been so strong a shift to the international system of classification that the second edition of Paterson's book published in 1963 simply mentions the Steinthal principles in two lines and then lists the international system with TNM (see below) designations as the only justifiable schema to use (reviewed in [Nachlas 1991]).

American pathologists Cushman *Davis* Haagensen (1900-1990) and Arthur *Purdy* Stout (1885-1967) reviewed 495 radical mastectomies performed during the period 1935 to 1942. They were able to identify clinical features of breast cancer that were associated with a 0% chance of a 5-year cure and a greater than 50% chance of a local recurrence [Haagensen and Stout 1943]. They recognized correlations between results and various clinical findings, identifying those with "grave signs" such as skin edema, ulceration, tumor fixation, axillary nodes larger than 2.5 cm, and arm edema. From these data, they constructed the Columbia Clinical Classification (CCC) system, one of the earliest attempts to match treatment to prognosis. CCC system staged breast cancers from A to D, with the letters A to C roughly corresponding to Steinthal's stages I to III:

- *Stage A*: No grave signs or clinically involved nodes.
- *Stage B:* Clinically involved but mobile axillary nodes less than 2.5 cm but no grave signs.
- *Stage C:* Any one of five grave signs.
- *Stage D:* All others with more advanced local disease and distant metastases.

Haagensen conceded that, although there may be some degree of imprecision in these clinical criteria, the various stages did show a significant spread in prognosis ranging from 73%, 58%, 24%, to 0% 5-year survivals. The CCC system was based on preoperative clinical assessment, and this was an important limitation. Frequently, inaccuracies in the original staging could be discovered after surgery. Thus this kind of staging could generate confuse information. This led Haagensen and Stout to develop the "triple biopsy" in the 1950's [Haagensen *et al.* 1963]. This examined tissue from the original breast mass, the internal mammary lymph nodes, and the nodes at the top of the axilla. Haagensen declined to perform radical mastectomy on women found to have cancer of the breast and in either of the other two areas. Believing that such patients were incurable, he sent them for palliative radiation therapy. The use of the triple biopsy substantially lowered the rate of operability to about 50%.

The Portmann Staging (POR) system was introduced in 1943 [Portmann 1943]. Ursus *Victor* Portmann (1887-1966) considered that classifications on histologic criteria were unsatisfactory, because of regional heterogeneity in tumors and because of variations between reporting pathologists. He was also aware of the shortcomings of classifications based only on clinical criteria, including that suggested by Steinthal, because they may not accurately reflect the presence or absence of metastases.

Starting in 1936, Portmann divided cases into three stages (or groups), on the basis of both clinical and pathologic criteria; in his 1943 paper, the third stage was subdivided to create a fourth stage having distant metastases detected clinically or by radiography, on presentation:

Stage I:

- Skin – not involved;
- Tumor – localized in the breast and movable;
- Metastases – none in axillary nodes or elsewhere.

Stage II:

- Skin – not involved;
- Tumor – localized in breast and movable;
- Metastases – few axillary lymph nodes involved, no other metastases.

Stage III:

- Skin – edematous; brawny red induration and inflammationnot obviously due to infection; extensive ulceration; multiple secondary nodules;
- Tumor – diffusely infiltrating breast; fixation of tumor or breast to chest wall; edema of breast
- Metastases: secondary tumors.

Stage IV:

- Skin – as in any other group or stage;
- Tumor – as in any other group or stage;
- Metastases – axillary and supraclavicular lymph nodes extensively involved and clinical or roentgenographic evidence of more distant metastases. (all this reviewed in [Weiss 2000])

The culmination of centuries of clinical observations is to be found in current classification and staging systems, based on the "TNM" classification advocated by French surgeon Pierre Denoix (1912-1990), of Institut Gustave Roussy, and his colleagues between 1943 and 1952 [Denoix 1944]. In 1947, Denoix summed up the results of studies on 25,000 case histories of patients with different cancers, in 55 designated, numbered groups. In a later publication [Denoix and Viollet 1950], the results of a multicenter study of 38,535 case histories were described which included the age of onset, localization, duration, evolution, histologic type and results of treatment. Introduction of the "TNM" staging system provided consistent descriptions of the anatomic extent of cancers at specific times in their development or clinical progression, in terms of the extent of the primary cancer (T), the absence, presence and extent of regional lymph node involvement (N), and the absence or presence of distant metastases (M).

The International Union Against Cancer (UICC) presented a clinical classification of breast cancer based on the TNM system in 1958 and the American Joint Committee on Cancer (AJCC) published a breast cancer staging system based on TNM in their first cancer staging manual in 1977. Since that time, regular revisions have been issued to reflect major advances in diagnosis and treatment. In the 1987 revision, differences between the AJCC and UICC versions of the TNM system were eliminated [Singletary and Connolly 2006].

The TNM system is the only staging system that is still in general use. It includes four classifications: clinical, pathologic, recurrence, and autopsy (in [Singletary and Connolly 2006]):

- Clinical classification (cTNM) is used to make local/regional treatment recommendations. It is based solely on evidence gathered before initial treatment of the primary tumor: physical examination, imaging studies (including mammography and ultrasound), and pathologic examination of the breast or other tissues obtained from biopsy as appropriate to establish the diagnosis of breast cancer.

- Pathologic classification (pTNM) is used to assess prognosis and to make recommendations for adjuvant treatment. It incorporates the results of clinical staging with evidence obtained from surgery and from detailed pathologic examination of the primary tumor, lymph nodes, and distant metastases (if present).
- Classification of a recurrent tumor (rTNM) is used when further treatment is needed for a tumor that has recurred after a disease-free interval and includes all information available at the time.
- Autopsy classification (aTNM) is used for cancers discovered after the death of a patient, when the cancer was not detected before death.

Additional descriptors are used for identification of special cases of cTNM or pTNM classifications, including the "m" prefix in cases with multiple tumors and the "y" prefix in cases where classification is performed during or following initial multimodality therapy (ie, neoadjuvant chemotherapy, radiation therapy, or both). Thus, ycTNM or ypTNM indicates the extent of tumor actually present at the time of that examination, rather than an estimate of tumor size before initiation of neoadjuvant therapy.

Table 3. TNM Classification for Breast Cancer

Classification	Definition
Primary tumor (T)	
TX	Primary tumor cannot be assessed
T0	No evidence of primary tumor
Tis	Carcinoma in situ
Tis (DCIS)	Ductal carcinoma in situ
Tis (LCIS)	Lobular carcinoma in situ
Tis (Paget)	Paget disease of the nipple with no tumor (Paget disease associated with a tumor is classified according to the size of the tumor.)
T1	Tumor <=2 cm in greatest dimension
T1mic	Microinvasion <=0.1 cm in greatest dimension
T1a	Tumor >0.1 cm but <=0.5 cm in greatest dimension

Classification	Definition
T1b	Tumor >0.5 cm but <=1 cm in greatest dimension
T1c	Tumor >1 cm but <=2 cm in greatest dimension
T2	Tumor >2 cm but <=5 cm in greatest dimension
T3	Tumor >5 cm in greatest dimension
T4	Tumor of any size with direct extension to chest wall or skin, only as described below
T4a	Extension to chest wall, not including pectoralis muscle
T4b	Edema (including peau d'orange) or ulceration of the skin of the breast, or satellite skin nodules confined to the same breast
T4c	Both T4a and T4b
T4d	Inflammatory carcinoma
Regional lymph nodes (N)	
NX	Regional lymph nodes cannot be assessed (eg, previously removed)
N0	No regional lymph node metastasis
N1	Metastasis in movable ipsilateral axillary lymph node(s)
N2	Metastases in ipsilateral axillary lymph nodes fixed or matted, or in clinically apparent[1] ipsilateral internal mammary nodes in the absence of clinically evident axillary lymph-node metastasis
N2a	Metastasis in ipsilateral axillary lymph nodes fixed to one another (matted) or to other structures
N2b	Metastasis only in clinically apparent[1] ipsilateral internal mammary nodes and in the absence of clinically evident axillary axillary lymph-node metastasis
N3	Metastasis in ipsilateral infraclavicular lymph node(s), or in clinically apparent[1] ipsilateral internal mammary lymph node(s) and in the presence of clinically evident axillary lymph-node metastasis; or metastasis in ipsilateral supraclavicular lymph node(s) with or without axillary or internal mammary lymph-node involvement

Table 3. (Continued)

Classification	Definition
N3a	Metastasis in ipsilateral infraclavicular lymph node(s) and axillary lymph node(s)
N3b	Metastasis in ipsilateral internal mammary lymph node(s) and axillary lymph node(s)
N3c	Metastasis in ipsilateral supraclavicular lymph node(s)
Regional lymph nodes (pN)[2]	
pNX	Regional lymph nodes cannot be assessed (eg, previously removed or not removed for pathologic study)
pN0	No regional lymph node metastasis histologically, no additional examination for isolated tumor cells[3]
pN0(i–)	No regional lymph node metastasis histologically, negative immunohistochemical staining
pN0(i+)	Isolated tumor cells identified histologically or by positive immunohistochemical staining, no cluster >0.2 mm
pN0(mol-)	No regional lymph-node metastasis histologically, negative molecular findings (reverse transcriptase/polymerase chain reaction)
pN0(mol+)	No regional lymph-node metastasis histologically, positive molecular findings (reverse transcriptase/polymerase chain reaction)
pN1	Metastasis in one to three axillary lymph nodes, and/or in internal mammary nodes with microscopic disease detected by sentinel lymph node dissection but not clinically apparent[1]
pN1mi	Micrometastasis (>0.2 mm, none >2.0 mm)
pN1a	Metastasis in one to three axillary lymph nodes
pN1b	Metastasis in internal mammary nodes with microscopic disease detected by sentinel lymph-node dissection but not clinically apparent[1]
pN1c	Metastasis in one to three axillary lymph nodes[4] and in internal mammary lymph nodes with microscopic disease detected by sentinel lymph-node dissection but not clinically apparent[1]
pN2	Metastasis in four to nine axillary lymph nodes, or in clinically apparent[1] internal mammary lymph nodes in the absence of axillary lymphnode metastasis

Classification	Definition
pN2a	Metastasis in four to nine axillary lymph nodes (at least one tumor deposit >2.0 mm)
pN2b	Metastasis in clinically apparent[1] internal mammary lymph nodes in the absence of axillary lymph-node metastasis
pN3	Metastasis in 10 or more axillary lymph nodes, or in infraclavicular lymph nodes, or in clinically apparent[1] ipsilateral internal mammary lymph nodes in the presence of one or more positive axillary lymph nodes; or in more than three axillary lymph nodes with clinically negative microscopic metastasis in internal mammary lymph nodes; or in ipsilateral supraclavicular lymph nodes
pN3a	Metastasis in 10 or more axillary lymph nodes (at least one tumor deposit >2.0 mm), or metastasis to the infraclavicular lymph nodes
pN3b	Metastasis in clinically apparent[1] ipsilateral internal mammary lymph nodes in the presence of one or more positive axillary lymph nodes; or in more than three axillary lymph nodes and in internal mammary lymph nodes with microscopic disease detected by sentinel lymph-node dissection but not clinically apparent[1]
pN3c	Metastasis in ipsilateral supraclavicular lymph nodes
Distant metastasis (M)	
MX	Distant metastasis cannot be assessed
M0	No distant metastasis
M1	Distant metastasis

(1) Clinically apparent is defined as detected by imaging studies (excluding lymphoscintigraphy) or by clinical examination.

(2) Classification is based on axillary lymph node dissection with or without sentinel lymph-node dissection. Classification based solely on sentinel lymph-node dissection without subsequent axillary lymph node dissection is designated (sn) for "sentinel node," such as pN0(i+)(sn).

(3) Isolated tumor cells are defined as single tumor cells or small cell clusters<=0.2 mm, usually detected only by immunohistochemical ormolecular methods but which may be verified on hematoxylin and eosin stains. Isolated tumor cells do not usually show evidence of metastaticactivity (eg, proliferation or stromal reaction).

(4) If associated with more than three positive axillary lymph nodes, the internal mammary nodes are classified as pN3b to reflect increased tumor burden.

Grading

Grading refers to the appearance of the cancer cells under the microscope.

In 1892, David von Hansemann proposed that the nuclear morphology of tumor cells might foretell their ultimate biological behavior [von Hansemann 1892]. This concept laid the foundation for a multitude of grading schemes that are in use today.

In 1925, Robert *Battey* Greenough (1871-1937) documented the relationship between histological grade and survival notably by assessing a series of morphological factors including gland formation, secretory vacuoles, cell size, nuclear size, pleomorphism, degree of hyperchromasia, and number of mitoses [Greenough 1925].

In 1928, David *Howard* Patey (1899-1977) and Robert *Wilfred* Scarff (1899-1970) highlighted the importance of tubular formation, variation in nuclear size, and hyperchromatism in histologic grading [Patey and Scarff 1928].

In 1933, Cushman *Davis* Haagensen (1900-1990) evaluated 15 histological features categorized under growth pattern, cell morphology, and the reaction of the surrounding stroma [Haagensen 1933].

In 1950, *Harris* Julian *Gaster* Bloom (1923-1989) divided tumors into low, moderate, or high-grade malignancies according to three features:

1) the extent of tubule formation;
2) nuclear hyperchromasia, pleomorphism and size, and
3) mitotic activity, and recognized a correlation between tumor grade and survival [Bloom 1950].

In 1957, Bloom and William *Worsley* Richardson (1915-2005) proposed a numerical scoring system to facilitate the grading effort [Bloom and Richardson 1957]. Each of the above three features was examined and given a score of 1, 2, or 3 for a total possible score ranging from 3 to 9. This system ("Bloom-Richardson" –BR- or Scarff-Bloom-Richardson" – SBR- system) was adopted by the World Health Organization (WHO) in 1968.

Nuclear grading is the cytological evaluation of tumor nuclei in comparison with the nuclei of normal mammary epithelial cells [Black and Speer 1957].

In 1975, Maurice *Meyer* Black (1918-1996) and colleagues [Black *et al.* 1975] concluded that nuclear morphology was the most significant prognostic factor. They proposed a five-grade (regularity of the nuclear outline, delicacy of the chromatin, nucleoli, and the presence and number of mitotic figures) nuclear grading system that was later (in 1980) reduced to three grades by Edwin Fisher and colleagues [Fisher *et al.* 1980].

In 1989, Viviane Le Doussal and colleagues created five grades based on nuclear pleomorphism and mitotic index. They omitted the degree of structural differentiation [Le Doussal *et al.* 1989].

• *Degree of tumor tubule formation*	*Score*
>75% of tumor cells arranged in tubules	1
>10% and <75%	2
<10%	3
• *Tumor mitotic activity* Microscope: low power scanning (X100), find most mitotically tumor area, proceed to high power (x400)	*Score*
<10 mitoses in 10 high-power fields	1
>10 and <20 mitoses	2
>20 mitoses per 10 high power fields	3
• *Nuclear grade of tumor cells*	Score
Cell nuclei are uniform in size and shape, relatively small, have dispersed chromatin patterns, and are without prominent nucleoli	1
Cell nuclei are somewhat pleomorphic, have nucleoli, and are intermediate size	2
Cell nuclei are relatively large, have prominent nucleoli or multiple nucleoli, coarse chromatin patterns, and vary in size and shape	3

The seven possible combined scores (from "3" to "9") are condensed into three Bloom-Richardson grades. The three grades then translate into well-differentiated (low grade), moderately differentiated (intermediate grade) and poorly differentiated (high grade).

Bloom-Richardson combined scores	Differentiation/BR Grade
3, 4, 5	Well-differentiated/low grade
6, 7	Moderately differentiated/intermediate grade
8, 9	Poorly differentiated/high grade

References

Black MM, Speer FD. Nuclear structure in cancer tissues. *Surg. Gynecol. Obstet.* 1957 Jul;105(1):97-102.

Black MM, Barclay THC, Hankey BF. Prognosis in breast cancer utilizing histologic characteristics of the primary tumor. *Cancer.* 1975 Dec;36(6):2048-55.

Bloom HJG.Prognosis in carcinoma of the breast. *Br. J. Cancer.* 1950 Sep;4(3):259-88.

Bloom HJG, Richardson WW. Histologic grading in breast cancer: a study of 1,409 cases of which 359 have been followed for 15 years. *Br. J. Cancer.* 1957 Sep;11(3):359-77..

Denoix PF. Sur l'organisation d'une statistique permanente du cancer. *Bull. Inst. Nat. Hyg.* (Paris) 1944;1:67–74.

Denoix PF and Viollet G. Six années d'enquête permanente cancer. *Bull. Inst. Nat. Hyg.* (Paris). 1950;5:44–84.

Elston CW, Ellis IO.Pathological prognostic factors in breast cancer. I. The value of histological grade in breast cancer: experience from a large study with long-term follow up. *Histopathology* 1991;19(5):403–410.

Fisher ER, Redmond C, Fisher B (1980) Histologic grading of breast cancer. *Pathol. Annu.* 1980;15(Pt 1):239-51.

Greenough RB. Varying degrees of malignancy in cancer of the breast. *J. Cancer Res.* 1925;9:452-63.

Haagensen CD. The basis for histologic grading of the breast. *Am. J. Cancer.* 1933;1:285–327.

Haagensen CD, Stout AP. Carcinoma of the breast: 11. Criteria of operability. *Ann. Surg* 1943;118:1032-51.

Haagensen CD, Cooley E, Kennedy CS, Miller E, Handley RS, Thackray AC, Butcher HR, Dahl-Iversen E, Tobiassen T, Williams IG, Curwen MP, Kaae S, Johansen H. Treatment of early mammary carcinoma: A cooperative international study. *Ann. Surg.* 1963 Feb;157(2):157-79.

Le Doussal V, Tubiana-Hulin M, Friedman S, Hacene K, Spyratos F, Brunet M. Prognostic value of histologic grade nuclear components of Scarff-Bloom-Richardson (SBR). An improved score modification based on a multivariate analysis of 1262 invasive ductal breast carcinomas. *Cancer.* 1989 Nov 1;64(9):1914-21.

Nachlas MM. Irrationality in the management of breast cancer. I. The staging system. *Cancer.* 1991 Aug 15;68(4):681-90.

Patey DH, Scarff RW. The position of histology in the prognosis of the breast. *Lancet* 1928;1:801–4.

Portmann UV. Clinical and pathologic criteria as a basis for classifying cases of primary cancer of the breast. *Cleve Clin. J. Med.* 1943;10:41-7.

Singletary SE, Connolly JL. Breast cancer staging: working with the sixth edition of the AJCC Cancer Staging Manual. *CA Cancer J. Clin.* 2006 Jan-Feb;56(1):37-47.

Steinthal K Zur Dauerheilung des Brustkrebses. *Beitr. Klin. Chir.* 1905;47:226-39.

Tawfik O, Kimler BF, Davis M, Stasik C, Lai SM, Mayo MS, Fan F, Donahue JK, Damjanov I, Thomas P, Connor C, Jewell WR, Smith H, Fabian CJ. Grading invasive ductal carcinoma of the breast: advantages of using automated proliferation index instead of mitotic count. *Virchows Arch.* 2007 Jun;450(6):627-36.

von Hansemann D. Uber assymetrische zelltheilung in epithelkrebsen und deren biologishe bedeutung. *Virchows Arch. Pathol. Anat.* 1890;119:299–326.

von Hansemann D. Ueber die Anaplasie der Geschwulstzellen und die asymmetrische mitose. *Virchows Arch. Pathol. Anat.* 1892;129:436–49.

Weiss L. Metastasis of cancer: a conceptual history from antiquity to the 1990s. *Cancer Metastasis Rev.* 2000;19(3-4):I-XI, 193-383.

Chapter 10

Twentieth Century and Beyond Breast Cancer Genetics

Abstract

Since the beginning of the 20th century, it was clear that many tumors were associated with chromosomal alterations. It was also suspected that tumor progression could be caused by a series of genetic changes. Progresses in genetic research and technical advances allowed the discovery of several oncogenes and tumor suppressor genes. Moreover, the hereditary nature of at least a fraction of breast cancer was confirmed by the identification of BRCA1 and BRCA2. Other genes, such as TP53, CHEK2, ATM, STK11/LKB and PTEN were associated to syndromes of which breast cancer may be a component. It is increasingly believed that most breast tumors have a multigenic origin.

In 1890, David von Hansemann (1858-1920) documented the occurrence of asymmetric nuclear divisions in a wide variety of human epithelial cancers. In these abnormal, but bipolar, divisions, he observed that a fraction of the chromosomes failed to segregate properly. von Hansemann hypothesized that aneuploidy was the cause of disordered growth observed in cancer [von Hansemann 1890].

In 1914, German geneticist Theodor Boveri (1862-1915), in agreement with von Hansemann's observations [Hardy and Zacharias 2005], proposed that a tumor typically originates from a single cell that has inherited a defined, but incorrectly combined, set of chromosomes [Boveri 1914; Boveri 2008]. He also suggested that tumors might result from genetic alterations that were not visible with a microscope because they did not involve entire chromosomes.

In 1916, Ernest *Edward* Tyzzer (1875–1965) was the first to use the term "somatic mutation". He provided experimental evidence for the link between somatic mutation and cancer in mice [Tyzzer 1916]. It is now clear that most cancers are somatic cells genetic diseases and that somatic mutation explains the clonal origin and the irreversibility of these cancers.

In 1925, American geneticist Thomas *Hunt* Morgan (1866-1945), working on *Drosophila* flies, suggested that gene mutation, rather than aneuploidy, was the major cause of abnormal phenotypes seen in cancer [Morgan and Bridges 1925]. Aneuploidy is now generally viewed as a consequence, and mutated genes as a cause of cancer, but the controversy is not closed as yet (see for instance [Li et al. 2000]).

The fact that genetic alterations can cause cancer was notably supported in 1927, when American geneticist and Nobel laureate Hermann *Joseph* Muller (1890–1967) demonstrated the mutagenic properties of X-rays [Muller 1927].

The observation that, in some tar-induced mouse tumors, tumor cells with a specific chromosome abnormality had additional chromosomal variations that differed from cell to cell provided support for the idea proposed in 1930 by Øjvind Winge (1886-1964) [Winge 1930] that a series of genetic changes could cause the stepwise clinical and biological progression of tumors.

In 1937, RP Martynova, of USSR (now Russia) established the definite role of hereditary factors in the predisposition to cancer of the breast in women [Martynova 1937]. A number of following studies consistently demonstrated a two- to three-fold increase in breast cancer risk in first degree relatives (mothers and sisters) of breast cancer patients. The role of heredity in genesis of cancers in general, and in particular in breast cancer, was reviewed by Oluf Jacobsen (b. 1906) in 1946. The author concluded that there are numerous inherited precancerous and cancerous conditions that are unequivocally linked with genetically determined genes. Among neoplasms with genetically transmitted genes, retinoblastoma, breast carcinoma, certain uterine and ovarian cancers, neurofibromatosis, and polyposis of the colon were listed (reviewed in [Hajdu 2006]).

In 1944, deoxyribonucleic acid (DNA) was found by Oswald *Theodore* Avery (1877-1955), Colin *Munro* MacLeod (1909-1972), and Maclyn McCarty (1911-2005) to be the basic genetic material [Avery *et al.* 1944].

In 1953, the most important discovery in biology during the 20th century was made, as James *Dewey* Watson (b. 1928) and Francis *Harry Compton* Crick (1916-2004), building on the work of Maurice *Hugh Frederick* Wilkins

(1916-2004) and Rosalind *Elsie* Franklin (1920-1958), elucidated the double helical structure of DNA [Watson and Crick 1953].

In 1953, Finnish born Carl *Olof* Nordling (1917-2007) proposed the multi-mutation theory of cancer. He suggested that the outbreak of cancer required the accumulation of six consecutive mutations [Nordling 1953]. In 1971, the theory was revived by Alfred *George* Knudson (b. 1922) and is now known as the "Knudson hypothesis". From studies on children with inherited or non-inherited ("sporadic") retinoblastoma, Knudson concluded that multiple "hits" to DNA were necessary to cause cancer. In inherited retinoblastoma, the first insult was inherited in the DNA, and any second insult would rapidly lead to cancer. In sporadic retinoblastoma, two "hits" had to take place before a tumor could develop, explaining the age difference. The theory has been extended to other cancers, including breast cancer.

In 1960, the first chromosome abnormality in cancer, the Philadelphia (Ph1) chromosome, was precisely described in chronic myelogenous leukemia by Peter *Carey* Nowell (b. 1928) and David Hungerford (1927-1993) [Nowell and Hungerford 1960].. It was later shown that the Ph1 chromosome arises from a translocation involving chromosomes 9 and 22. This translocation results in the formation of a hybrid gene (bcr/abl), which, in turn, codes for a hybrid protein that predisposes cells to become leukemic. It is now known that most cancer cells show karyotypic changes with a variety of chromosomal abnormalities. This is also observed in breast cancer [Devilee and Cornelisse 1994; Lacroix *et al.* 2004]. The discovery of Nowell and colleagues supported Boveri's theory and the general opinion that most human tumors resulted from chromosome alterations and that the more advanced a neoplasm was the more extensive the chromosome alterations were likely to be. However, because no consistent chromosome abnormality other than the Philadelphia chromosome had been associated with a specific type of tumor, it was thought that the chromosome alterations were probably the result, rather than the cause, of the neoplasm. Furthermore, although some investigators thought that the chromosome abnormalities had an important role in tumor progression, others believed that they had no basic role in tumorigenesis.

In 1961, South African biologist Sidney Brenner (b. 1927) and Francis Crick established that groups of three nucleotide bases, or codons, are used to specify individual amino acids. The genetic code of nucleotide triplets was worked out in final detail in 1966 and paved the way for the molecular analysis of gene damage.

Still in 1961, Sydney Brenner, French biologist Francois Jacob (b. 1920) and American geneticist and molecular biologist Matthew Meselson (b. 1930) showed that ribosomes are the site of protein synthesis and that RNA carries messages from the DNA to the ribosome.

The production of heritable changes in gene expression is the driving force in the development and progression of breast cancer. Such changes can result from mutations or from epigenetic events such as hypoacetylation of histones and hypermethylation of DNA. These epigenetic alterations appear as major determinants of chromatin structure. Chromatin structure is a primary regulator of gene transcription. Cancer cells frequently contain both mutated genes and genes with altered expression due to one or more epigenetic mechanisms.

In 1964, Vincent *George* Allfrey (1921-2002), Alfred *Ezra* Mirsky (1900-1974) and colleagues proposed that histone acetylation was associated with transcriptional activity in eukaryotic cells [Allfrey *et al.* 1964]. Acetylation (by histone acetyltransferases or HAT) neutralizes the charge of the histones and generates a more open DNA conformation. Transcription factors then have access to the DNA and expression of the corresponding genes is promoted. Deacetylation (by histone deacetylases or HDAC) locks up the DNA in nucleosomes thereby preventing transcription. This implied the possibility of a role for histone acetylation in cancer. The importance of acetylation for the regulation of gene expression and gene silencing in cancer was, however, realized only many years later. The potential anticancer activities of histone deacetylase (HDAC) inhibitors are still under examination.

DNA methylation is a covalent modification of the C5 position in cytosine. This methylation pattern is stably maintained at CpG dinucleotides by a family of DNA methyltransferases (DNMT) that recognize semi-methylated CpG dinucleotides after DNA replication (review by [Mielnicki *et al.* 2001]). Regulatory CpG islands are present at the 5' ends of most housekeeping and some tissue-specific genes in the mammalian genome. There are approximately 45,000 CpG islands and these are generally unmethylated in normal cells. Hypermethylation of CpG dinucleotides within regions of the gene promoter and/or intronic sequences is associated with transcriptional repression. DNA hypo-methylation was identified as a characteristic of cancer cells in 1983 [Feinberg and Vogelstein 1983]. However, many specific genes have been found hypermethylated in breast tumors but not in normal breast tissues (see notably in [Lacroix *et al.* 2004]).

The potential anticancer activities of and DNA methyltransferase (DNMT) inhibitors have been extensively studied in recent years.

DNMT inhibitors, such as 5-aza-cytidine (5-aza-CR) and 5-aza-2'-deoxycytidine (5-aza-CdR) are also widely studied because DNA hypomethylation induces the re-activation of tumor suppressor genes that are silenced by methylation-mediated mechanisms.

In 1969, Robert *Joseph* Huebner (1914-1998) and George Todaro (b. 1937) proposed the oncogene hypothesis [Huebner and Todaro 1969]. An oncogene is a gene that has the potential to make a cell become cancerous. Oncogenes arise from normal genes, or proto-oncogenes, by mutation or by increased expression. Most proto-oncogenes control growth and differentiation of cells. The first oncogene, src, was discovered in 1976 by Dominique Stéhelin (b. 1943), John *Michael* Bishop (b. 1936) and Harold *Elliot* Varmus (b. 1939).

In 1969, Frederick Pei Li (b. 1940) and Joseph Francis Fraumeni, Jr (b. 1933) [Li and Fraumeni 1969] described breast cancer in association with soft-tissue sarcomas, leukemia, and lymphoma in four families. Subsequently, the "Li-Fraumeni syndrome" was characterized by early age of onset of breast cancer in concert with sarcoma, brain, lung, leukemia, lymphoma, and adrenal cortical carcinoma. It is also known as the SBLA syndrome [Lynch *et al.* 1978]. In 1990, germ-line mutations in the TP53 tumor suppressor gene (see below) were associated to the Li-Fraumeni syndrome [Malkin *et al.* 1990; Srivastava *et al.* 1990]. However, such germ-line alterations may account for only 1% of breast cancers diagnosed before the age of 35. Research today is looking at ways of targeting p53 in anti-cancer therapy, for example by restoring its function in cancer cells.

in situ hybridization, a technique that allows nucleic acid sequences to be examined inside cells or on chromosomes was first described in 1969 by Joseph Grafton Gall (b. 1928) and Mary-Lou Pardue (b. 1933) [Gall and Pardue 1969]. These authors used radioactive probes. The first molecular cytogenetic experiment on human chromosomes was performed in 1986, when Daniel Pinkel, Joseph William Gray and colleagues [Pinkel *et al.* 1986] used fluorescent in situ hybridization ("FISH"). First FISH studies on breast cancer were published in the early 1990's.

In 1976, German virologist Harald zur Hausen (b. 1936) proposed that human papillomavirus (HPV) was the cause of cervical cancer. In 1983 and 1984, zur Hausen discovered HPV DNA in cervical cancer tumors, proving his theory. Almost 20% of cancers worldwide are attributable to infectious diseases, and prophylactic vaccination against the infecting organisms may offer significant protection against the related cancers [Parkin 2006]. The search for an infectious etiology for breast cancer has been going on for many years, with most research centering on papillomavirus, Epstein-Barr virus, and a human equivalent of mouse mammary tumor virus (see chapter 12) (reviewed by [Singletary 2007]). However, the evidence of a viral etiology, while suggested by these works, remains largely descriptive and indirect. It is likely that, if such a relationship exists, then it will be much more complex than the simple relationship observed for such conditions as influenza [Singletary 2007].

In 1979, murine tumor protein 53 (p53) was identified. Human p53 and its corresponding gene (TP53) were found in the following years. In 1989, TP53 was found to be a tumor suppressor gene [Finlay et al. 1989]. Most tumor suppressor genes code for enzymes that control DNA transcription, DNA repair, and other functions. Damage to these genes, whether by a chemical carcinogen, virus, or ionizing radiation, can lead to mutations and malignancy TP53 has a role in preventing DNA mutation, which can lead to cancer. It becomes active when DNA damage is detected. TP53 is the most frequently mutated gene in human cancer (approximately 50% of cases). It is less-frequently altered in breast cancer (20-25% of cases) [Lacroix et al. 2006], but TP53 germ-line mutations have been associated to the Li-Fraumeni syndrome (see above) [Lacroix and Leclercq 2005].

In 1985, an oncogene was independently discovered by three teams and simultaneously named HER-2/neu [Coussens et al. 1985] and c-erbB2 [Semba et al. 1985; King et al. 1985]. HER-2/neu is related to, but distinct from, the epidermal growth factor receptor (EGFR). In 1987, the first data demonstrating a link between overexpression of HER2/neu and the progression of breast cancer were published by Dennis *Joseph* Slamon (b. 1948) and colleagues [Slamon et al. 1987]. Later studies showed that the aggressiveness of some breast cancers was linked to the amplification of the HER-2 gene (named *ERBB2*). An antibody directed against the HER2 protein was developed (trastuzumab, see chapter 8) and was shown to slow or block the progression of some breast cancer. Trastuzumab is now FDA-approved and commercialized.

In 1990, linkage for early onset site-specific breast cancer on chromosome 17q was identified [Hall et al. 1990]. Shortly thereafter, in 1991, linkage to this same locus (17q12-q23), in concert with ovarian cancer in the hereditary breast-ovarian cancer (HBOC) syndrome was shown [Narod et al. 1991]. The gene at locus 17q12-q23, named BRCA1, was cloned in 1994 [Miki et al. 1994]. BRCA1, is considered to be responsible for 2% to 4% of all breast cancer [Lacroix and Leclercq 2005]. In 1995, a second breast cancer gene was shown to be linked to chromosome 13q [Wooster et al. 1994], and was identified and named BRCA2 [Wooster et al. 1995]. Like TP53, BRCA1 and BRCA2 are tumor suppressor genes. Their discovery contributed greatly to the understanding of hereditary breast cancer.Genetic testing for BRCA1 and BRCA2 abnormalities is now available.

In 1992, comparative genomic hybridization (CGH) was introduced [Kallioniemi *et al.* 1992]. This molecular cytogenetic technique allows the detection of DNA losses or gains larger than 10 megabases in tumors. First CGH results in breast cancer were soon obtained [Kallioniemi *et al.* 1994]. For a review on DNA gains and losses in breast cancer, see [Lacroix *et al.* 2004] or [Climent *et al.* 2007].

In 1995, the first DNA microarray chip was constructed and used to measure global gene expression levels in plants [Schena *et al.* 1995]. Microarray use to study breast cancer has flourished since the early 2000's. Major information has been obtained, particularly in classifying breast tumors in different subtypes ("luminal-like", "basal-like", "ERBB2") and risk groups (for more data about microarray studies on breast cancer, see for instance [Sorlie *et al.* 2003; Lacroix and Leclercq 2004; Lacroix *et al.* 2004; Cianfrocca and Gradishar 2009]. Combining gene-expression data with other genomic information and the use of sophisticated bioinformatic tools enables the discovery of potential new targets for treatment, and is helpful for high-throughput drug screening and for designing new classes of drugs for targeted therapy (for a review, see [Foekens *et al.* 2008]).

In 1998, tissue microarrays were introduced and immediately used to analyze breast tumors [Kononen *et al.* 1998; for a review, see Brennan *et al.* 2007]. With this technique hundreds of cylindrical tissue biopsies from individual tumors can be distributed in a single tumor tissue microarray. Sections of the microarray provide targets for parallel*in situ* detection of DNA, RNA and protein targets in each specimen on the array, and consecutive sections allow the rapid analysis of hundreds of molecular markers in the same set of specimens [Korsching *et al.* 2002; Callagy *et al.* 2003; van der Vegt *et al.* 2009].Five to ten percent of all breast cancers are clearly inherited, the remaining being considered as "sporadic". While a majority of inherited cases have been attributed to mutations in BRCA1 or BRCA2, no BRCA3 has been found as yet. Part of the "non-BRCA1/non-BRCA2" lesions may be associated to rare syndromes, of which breast cancer is only one component. This is the case for TP53 (Li-Fraumeni syndrome, see above), CHEK2, ATM, STK11/LKB and PTEN [Lacroix *et al.* 2005?]. Indeed, in 2003, hereditary breast and colorectal cancer (HBCC) was associated to the 1100delC variant of the cell cycle checkpoint kinase *CHEK2* gene [Meijers-Heijboer *et al.* 2003]. Previously, germ-line mutations in ATM (11q22-23) had been associated with Ataxia-Telangiectasia [Savitsky *et al.* 1995], a disordercharacterized by cerebellar ataxia, telangiectasias, immune defects, and a predisposition to malignancy. Breast cancer is observed in ATM heterozygotes.Peutz-Jeghers syndrome is clinically characterized by mucocutaneous melanocytic pigmentation, intestinal hamartomatous polyposis and a significantly increased risk of developing cancer. It was association with STK11/LKB (19p13.3) in 1998 [Jenne et al. 1998; Hemminki et al. 1998]. In 1997 was demonstrated the association between germ-line mutations in PTEN (10q23) and Cowden's disease, which in addition to breast cancer, includes thyroid cancer and the presence of multiple hamartomas in the skin and gastrointestinal tract. [Liaw et al. 1997]. Somatic mutations in PTEN are quite rare in breast cancer: it is primarily responsible for 1 in a 1000 cases of breast cancer. Other BRCAx tumors, as well as many sporadic carcinomas, are increasingly believed to have a "multigenic" origin, thus resulting from the expression of weakly penetrant but highly prevalent mutations in various genes. For instance, polymorphism has been identified in genes associated to the metabolism of various potentially toxic compounds; the estrogen pathway; the DNA damage response pathways; other processes,for which additional data are provided in Table 4. Sequence variants of these genes that are relatively common in the population may be associated with a small to moderate increased relative risk for breast cancer. However, combinations of such variants could lead to multiplication effects and constitute the molecular bases for the development of BRCAx hereditary breast cancers. Sporadic cancers likely result from the complex interplay between the expression of low penetrance gene(s) ("risk variants") and environmental factors.

Table 4. Low penetrance genes. At least one allelic variant has been associated with increased breast cancer risk

Unigene Name	Complete protein name	Protein Function	Locus
NAT1	N-acetyl transferase 1	Detoxification of arylamines	8p22
NAT2	N-acetyl transferase 2	Detoxification of arylamines	8p22
GSTM1	Glutathione S-transferase M1	Detoxification of xenobiotics	1p13.3
GSTP1	Glutathione S-transferase P1	Detoxification of xenobiotics	11q13
GSTT1	Glutathione S-transferase T1	Detoxification of xenobiotics	22q11.2
CYP1A1	Cytochrome P450, family 1, subfamily A, member 1	Metabolism of potentially toxic compounds (including various aryl hydrocarbons)	15q22-q24

Unigene Name	Complete protein name	Protein Function	Locus
CYP1B1	Cytochrome P450, family 1, subfamily B, member 1	Metabolism of potentially toxic compounds (including various aryl hydrocarbons)	2p22-p21
CYP2D6	Cytochrome P450, family 2, subfamily D, member 6	Metabolism of potentially toxic compounds (debrisoquine, codeine,...)	22q13.1
COMT	Catechol O-methyltransferase	Metabolism of estrogens	22q11.2
CYP17A1	Cytochrome P450, family 17, subfamily A, member 1	Metabolism of estrogens	10q24.3
CYP19A1	Cytochrome P450, family 19, subfamily A, member 1	Metabolism of estrogens	15q21.1
ESR1	Oestrogen receptor	Response to estrogens	6q25.1
NCOA3 (AIB1)	Nuclear co-activator 3	Steroid receptor co-activation	20q12
PGR	Progesterone receptor	Response to estrogens	11q22-23
UGT1A1	Uridine diphospho-glucuronosyltransferase	Metabolism of estrogens	2q37
CHEK2	Checkpoint kinase 2	DNA damage response and repair	22q12.1
XRCC1	X-ray repair, complementing defective, in Chinese hamster, 1	DNA damage response and repair	19q13.2
XRCC3	X-ray repair, complementing defective, in Chinese hamster, 3	DNA damage response and repair	14q32.3
XRCC5	X-ray repair, complementing defective, in Chinese hamster, 5	DNA damage response and repair	2q35
AR	Androgen receptor	Response to androgens	Xq11-q12
HRAS	V-HA-Ras Harvey rat sarcoma viral oncogene homolog	Signaling	11p15.5
VDR	Vitamin D receptor	Response to vitamin D	12q12-q14

It must be noted, however, that the suspected impact of most of these variants on breast cancer risk should, in most cases, be confirmed in large populations studies. Indeed, low penetrance genes cannot be easily tracked through families, as is true for dominant high-risk genes.

In 2001, the discovery of microRNAs was reported [Lagos-Quintana *et al.* 2001]. They are a class of small (18-27 nucleotides) regulatory RNAs that influence the stability and translational efficiency of target mRNAs. Alterations in miRNA expression have been associated with a number of biological processes, including breast cancer [Iorio *et al.* 2005; Khoshnaw *et al.* 2009]

References

Allfrey VG, Faulkner R, Mirsky AE. Acetylation and methylation of histones and their possible role in the regulation of RNA synthesis. *Proc. Natl. Acad. Sci. U S A*. 1964 May;51:786-94.

Avery OT, Macleod CM, McCarty M. Studies on the chemical natureof the substance inducing transformation of pneumococcal types: induction of transformation by a desoxyribonucleic acid fraction isolated from Pneumococcus type III. J Exp Med. 1944 Feb 1;79(2):137-158.

Boveri T. *ZurFrage der Entwicklung maligner Tumoren.* (Jena, Gustav Fisher Verlag) 1914: 1-64

Boveri T. Concerning the Origin of Malignant Tumours by Theodor Boveri. Translated and annotated by Henry Harris. *Journal of Cell Science* 121, Supplement 1, 1-84 (2008).

Brennan DJ, Kelly C, Rexhepaj E, Dervan PA, Duffy MJ, Gallagher WM. Contribution of DNA and tissue microarray technology to the identification and validation of biomarkers and personalised medicine in breast cancer. *Cancer Genomics Proteomics*. 2007 May-Jun;4(3):121-34.

Callagy G, Cattaneo E, Daigo Y, Happerfield L, Bobrow LG, Pharoah PD, Caldas C. Molecular classification of breast carcinomas using tissue microarrays. *Diagn. Mol. Pathol*. 2003 Mar;12(1):27-34.

Cianfrocca M, Gradishar W. New molecular classifications of breast cancer. *CA Cancer J. Clin*. 2009 Sep-Oct;59(5):303-13.

Climent J, Garcia JL, Mao JH, Arsuaga J, Perez-Losada J. Characterization of breast cancer by array comparative genomic hybridization. *Biochem. Cell Biol*. 2007 Aug;85(4):497-508.

Coussens L, Yang-Feng TL, Liao YC, Chen E, Gray A, McGrath J, Seeburg PH, Libermann TA, Schlessinger J, Francke U, et al. Tyrosine kinase receptor with extensive homology to EGF receptor shares chromosomal location with neu oncogene. *Science.* 1985 Dec 6;230(4730):1132-9.

Devilee P, Cornelisse CJ. Somatic genetic changes in human breast cancer. *Biochim. Biophys. Acta.* 1994 Dec 30;1198(2-3):113-30.

Feinberg AP, Vogelstein B. 1983. Hypomethylation distinguishes genes of some human cancers from their normal counterparts. *Nature* 301:89–92.

Finlay CA, Hinds PW, Levine AJ. The p53 proto-oncogene can act as a suppressor of transformation. *Cell.* 1989 Jun 30;57(7):1083-93.

Foekens JA, Wang Y, Martens JW, Berns EM, Klijn JG. The use of genomic tools for the molecular understanding of breast cancer and to guide personalized medicine. *Drug Discov. Today.* 2008 Jun;13(11-12):481-7.

Gall JG, Pardue ML. Formation and detection of RNA-DNA hybrid molecules in cytological preparations. *Proc. Natl. Acad. Sci. U S A.* 1969 Jun;63(2):378-83.

Hajdu SI. Thoughts about the cause of cancer. *Cancer.* 2006 Apr 15;106(8):1643-9.

Hall JM, Lee MK, Newman B, Morrow JE, Anderson LA, Huey B, King MC. Linkage of early-onset breast cancer to chromosome 17q21. *Science.* 1990 Dec 21;250(4988):1684-9.

Hardy PA, Zacharias H. Reappraisal of the Hansemann-Boveri hypothesis on the origin of tumors. *Cell Biol. Int.* 2005 Dec;29(12):983-92.

Hemminki A, Markie D, Tomlinson I, Avizienyte E, Roth S, Loukola A, Bignell G, Warren W, Aminoff M, Höglund P, Järvinen H, Kristo P, Pelin K, Ridanpää M, Salovaara R, Toro T, Bodmer W, Olschwang S, Olsen AS, Stratton MR, de la Chapelle A, Aaltonen LA. A serine/threonine kinase gene defective in Peutz-Jeghers syndrome. *Nature.* 1998 Jan 8;391(6663):184-7.

Huebner RJ, Todaro GJ. Oncogenes of RNA tumor viruses as determinants of cancer. *Proc. Natl. Acad. Sci. U S A.* 1969 Nov;64(3):1087-94.

Iorio MV, Ferracin M, Liu CG, Veronese A, Spizzo R, Sabbioni S, Magri E, Pedriali M, Fabbri M, Campiglio M, Ménard S, Palazzo JP, Rosenberg A, Musiani P, Volinia S, Nenci I, Calin GA, Querzoli P, Negrini M, Croce CM. MicroRNA gene expression deregulation in human breast cancer. *Cancer Res.* 2005 Aug 15;65(16):7065-70.

Jenne DE, Reimann H, Nezu J, Friedel W, Loff S, Jeschke R, Müller O, Back W, Zimmer M. Peutz-Jeghers syndrome is caused by mutations in a novel serine threonine kinase. *Nat. Genet.* 1998 Jan;18(1):38-43.

Kallioniemi A, Kallioniemi OP, Sudar D, Rutovitz D, Gray JW, Waldman F, Pinkel D. Comparative genomic hybridization for molecular cytogenetic analysis of solid tumors. *Science.* 1992 Oct 30;258(5083):818-21.

Kallioniemi A, Kallioniemi OP, Piper J, Tanner M, Stokke T, Chen L, Smith HS, Pinkel D, Gray JW, Waldman FM. Detection and mapping of amplified DNA sequences in breast cancer by comparative genomic hybridization. *Proc. Natl. Acad. Sci. U S A.* 1994 Mar 15;91(6):2156-60.

King CR, Kraus MH, Aaronson SA. Amplification of a novel v-erbB-related gene in a human mammary carcinoma. *Science.* 1985 Sep 6;229(4717):974-6.

Kononen J, Bubendorf L, Kallioniemi A, Bärlund M, Schraml P, Leighton S, Torhorst J, Mihatsch MJ, Sauter G, Kallioniemi OP. Tissue microarrays for high-throughput molecular profiling of tumor specimens. *Nat. Med.* 1998 Jul;4(7):844-7.

Korsching E, Packeisen J, Agelopoulos K, Eisenacher M, Voss R, Isola J, van Diest PJ, Brandt B, Boecker W, Buerger H. Cytogenetic alterations and cytokeratin expression patterns in breast cancer: integrating a new model of breast differentiation into cytogenetic pathways of breast carcinogenesis. *Lab. Invest.* 2002 Nov;82(11):1525-33.

Khoshnaw SM, Green AR, Powe DG, Ellis IO. MicroRNA involvement in the pathogenesis and management of breast cancer. *J. Clin. Pathol.* 2009 May;62(5):422-8.

Lacroix M, Toillon RA, Leclercq G. Stable 'portrait' of breast tumors during progression: data from biology, pathology and genetics. Endocr Relat *Cancer.* 2004 Sep;11(3):497-522.

Lacroix M, Leclercq G. The "portrait" of hereditary breast cancer. *BreastCancer Res. Treat.* 2005 Feb;89(3):297-304.

Lacroix M, Toillon RA, Leclercq G. p53 and breast cancer, an update. Endocr Relat *Cancer.* 2006 Jun;13(2):293-325.

Lagos-Quintana M, Rauhut R, Lendeckel W, Tuschl T. Identification of novel genes coding for small expressed RNAs. *Science.* 2001 Oct 26;294(5543):853-8.

Liaw D, Marsh DJ, Li J, Dahia PL, Wang SI, Zheng Z, Bose S, Call KM, Tsou HC, Peacocke M, Eng C, Parsons R. Germline mutations of the PTEN gene in Cowden disease, an inherited breast and thyroid cancer syndrome. *Nat. Genet.* 1997 May;16(1):64-7.

Li FP, Fraumeni JF Jr. Soft-tissue sarcomas, breast cancer, and other neoplasms. A familial syndrome? *Ann. Intern. Med.* 1969 Oct;71(4):747-52.

Li R, Sonik A, Stindl R, Rasnick D, Duesberg P. Aneuploidy vs. gene mutation hypothesis of cancer: recent study claims mutation but is found to support aneuploidy. *Proc. Natl. Acad. Sci. U S A.* 2000 Mar 28;97(7):3236-41.

Lynch HT, Mulcahy GM, Harris RE, Guirgis HA, Lynch JF. Genetic and pathologic findings in a kindred with hereditary sarcoma, breast cancer, brain tumors, leukemia, lung, laryngeal, and adrenal cortical carcinoma. *Cancer.* 1978 May;41(5):2055-64.

Malkin D, Li FP, Strong LC, Fraumeni JF Jr, Nelson CE, Kim DH, Kassel J, Gryka MA, Bischoff FZ, Tainsky MA, et al. Germ line p53 mutations in a familial syndrome of breast cancer, sarcomas, and other neoplasms. *Science.* 1990 Nov 30;250(4985):1233-8.

Martynova RP. Studies in the genetics of human neoplasms. Cancer of the breast, based on 201 family histories. *Am. J. Cancer* 1937;29:530–540.

Meijers-Heijboer H, Wijnen J, Vasen H, Wasielewski M, Wagner A, Hollestelle A, Elstrodt F, van den Bos R, de Snoo A, Fat GT, Brekelmans C, Jagmohan S, Franken P, Verkuijlen P, van den Ouweland A, Chapman P, Tops C, Möslein G, Burn J, Lynch H, Klijn J, Fodde R, Schutte M. The CHEK2 1100delC mutation identifies families with a hereditary breast and colorectal cancer phenotype. *Am. J. Hum. Genet.* 2003 May;72(5):1308-14.

Mielnicki LM, Asch HL, Asch BB. Genes, chromatin, and breast cancer: an epigenetic tale. *J. Mammary Gland Biol. Neoplasia.* 2001 Apr;6(2):169-82.

Miki Y, Swensen J, Shattuck-Eidens D, Futreal PA, Harshman K, Tavtigian S, Liu Q, Cochran C, Bennett LM, Ding W, Bell R, Rosenthal J, Hussey C, Tran T, McClureM, Frye C, Hattier T, Phelps R, Haugen-Strano A, Katcher H, Yakumo K, Gholami Z, Shaffer D, Stone S, Bayer S, Wray C, Bogden R, Dayananth P, Ward J, Tonin P, Narod S, Bristow PK, Norris FH, Helvering L, Morrison P, Rosteck P, Lai M, Barrett JC, Lewis C, Neuhausen S, Cannon-Albright L, Goldgar D, Wiseman R, Kamb A, Skolnick MH. A strong candidate for the breast and ovarian cancer susceptibility gene BRCA1. *Science.* 1994 Oct 7;266(5182):66-71.

Morgan TH, Bridges CB, Sturtevant AH. The genetics of Drosophila. *Bibliogr. Genet* 1925;2:3–262.

Muller HJ. Artificial transmutation of the gene. *Science.* 1927 Jul 22;66(1699):84-7.

Narod SA, Feunteun J, Lynch HT, Watson P, Conway T, Lenoir GM. Familial breast-ovarian cancer locus on chromosome 17q12-q23. *Lancet.* 1991 Jul 13;338(8759):82-3.

Nordling CO. A new theory on cancer-inducing mechanism. *Br. J. Cancer.* 1953 Mar;7(1):68-72.

Nowell PC, Hungerford DA. Chromosome studies on normal and leukemic human leukocytes. *J. Natl. Cancer Inst.* 1960 Jul;25:85-109.

Parkin DM. The global health burden of infection-associated cancers in the year 2002. *Int. J. Cancer.* 2006 Jun 15;118(12):3030-44.

Pinkel D, Straume T, Gray JW. Cytogenetic analysis using quantitative, high-sensitivity, fluorescence hybridization. *Proc. Natl. Acad. Sci. U S A.* 1986 May;83(9):2934-8.

Savitsky K, Bar-Shira A, Gilad S, Rotman G, Ziv Y, Vanagaite L, Tagle DA, Smith S, Uziel T, Sfez S, Ashkenazi M, Pecker I, Frydman M, Harnik R, Patanjali SR, Simmons A, Clines GA, Sartiel A, Gatti RA, Chessa L, Sanal O, Lavin MF, Jaspers NG, Taylor AM, Arlett CF, Miki T, Weissman SM, Lovett M, Collins FS, Shiloh Y. A single ataxia telangiectasia gene with a product similar to PI-3 kinase. *Science.* 1995 Jun 23;268(5218):1749-53.

Schena M, Shalon D, Davis RW, Brown PO. Quantitative monitoring of gene expression patterns with a complementary DNA microarray. *Science.* 1995 Oct 20;270(5235):467-70.

Semba K, Kamata N, Toyoshima K, Yamamoto T. A v-erbB-related protooncogene, c-erbB-2, is distinct from the c-erbB-1/epidermal growth factor-receptor gene and is amplified in a human salivary gland adenocarcinoma. Proc Natl Acad Sci U S A. 1985 Oct;82(19):6497-501.

Singletary SE. Multidisciplinary frontiers in breast cancer management: a surgeon's perspective. *Cancer.* 2007 Mar 15;109(6):1019-29.

Slamon DJ, Clark GM, Wong SG, Levin WJ, Ullrich A, McGuire WL. Human breast cancer: correlation of relapse and survival with amplification of the HER-2/neu oncogene. *Science.* 1987 Jan 9;235(4785):177-82.

Sorlie T, Tibshirani R, Parker J, Hastie T, Marron JS, Nobel A, Deng S, Johnsen H, Pesich R, Geisler S, Demeter J, Perou CM, Lønning PE, Brown PO, Børresen-Dale AL, Botstein D. Repeated observation of breast tumor subtypes in independent gene expression data sets. *Proc. Natl. Acad. Sci. U S A.* 2003 Jul 8;100(14):8418-23.

Srivastava S, Zou ZQ, Pirollo K, Blattner W, Chang EH. Germ-line transmission of a mutated p53 gene in a cancer-prone family with Li-Fraumeni syndrome. *Nature.* 1990 Dec 20-27;348(6303):747-9.

Tyzzer EE. Tumor immunity. *J. Cancer Res.* 1916;1:125–56.

van der Vegt B, de Bock GH, Hollema H, Wesseling J. Microarray methods to identify factors determining breast cancer progression: potentials, limitations, and challenges. *Crit. Rev. Oncol. Hematol.* 2009 Apr;70(1):1-11.

von Hansemann D. Über asymmetrische Zellteilung in Epithelkrebsen und deren biologische Bedeutung. *Virchows Archiv. für Pathologische Anatomie* 1890;119:299–326.

Watson JD, Crick FH. Molecular structure of nucleic acids; a structure for deoxyribose nucleic acid. *Nature.* 1953 Apr 25;171(4356):737-8.

Winge Ø. Zytologische untersuchungen Über die natur maligner Tumoren. II.: Teerkarzinome bei Mauren. Z. Zellforsch. 1930;10:683.

Wooster R, Neuhausen SL, Mangion J, Quirk Y, Ford D, Collins N, Nguyen K, Seal S, Tran T, Averill D, Fields P, Marshall G, Narod S, Lenoir GM, Lynch H, Feunteun J, Devilee P, Cornelisse CJ, Menko FH, Daly PA, Ormiston W, McManus R, Pye C, Lewis CM, Cannon-Albright LA, Peto J, Ponder BAJ, Klolnick MH, Easton DF, Goldgar DE, Stratton MR. Localization of a breast cancer susceptibility gene, BRCA2, to chromosome 13q12-13. *Science.* 1994 Sep 30;265(5181):2088-90.

Wooster R, Bignell G, Lancaster J, Swift S, Seal S, Mangion J, Collins N, Gregory S, Gumbs C, Micklem G, Barfoot R, Hamoudi R, Patel S, Rice C, Biggs P, Hashim T, Smith A, Connor F, Arason A, Gudmundsson J, Ficenec D, Kelsell D, Ford D, Tonin P, Bishop DT, Spurr NK, Ponder BAJ, Eeles R, Peto J, Devilee P, Cornelisse C, Lynch H, Narod S, Lenoir G, Egilsson V, Bjork Barkadottir R, Easton DF, Bentley DR, Futreal PA, Ashworth A, Stratton MR. Identification of the breast cancer susceptibility gene BRCA2. *Nature.* 1995 Dec 21-28;378(6559):789-92.

Chapter 11

Twentieth Century and Beyond Breast Cancer Imaging and Detection

Abstract

Imaging is now an essential technique to identify breast tumors and to accompany breast cancer therapy. Imaging is also increasingly used for breast biopsies. Widely used since the 1970's, mammography, the most important advance in the 20th century in the clinical detection of cancer,is still the method of choice to screen women who show no signs or symptoms of the disease (prevention). Additional approved imaging methods frequently used as adjunct to mammography are ultrasonography and magnetic resonance imaging (MRI). Throughout the 20th century, a series of other approaches have been tried, including optical imaging, thermography or elastography. Promising techniques are positron emission tomography (PET), (99mTc) sestamibi scintimammography and electrical impedance tomography (EIT).

Mammography

Probably the earliest exploration of mammography was reported by German surgeon Albert Salomon (1883-1976). He used X-ray photography on about 3000 removed breast samples. He was able to distinguish highly infiltrating carcinoma from circumscribed carcinoma and demonstrated features like malignancy-associated breast calcifications and occult cancer [Salomon 1913].

In 1926, Stafford *Leak* Warren (1896-1981) developed a method to obtain stereoscopic films of breasts before surgery. He introduced X-rays for diagnostic examination of the breast and reported his observations a few years after [Warren 1930; Fray and Warren 1932]. From these studies, it was concluded that "most of the gross pathological changes were as readily identified in stereoscopic roentgenograms as they are in the gross specimen at biopsy or autopsy".

In 1938, Jacob Gershon-Cohen (1899-1971) and Albert Strickler (1886-1953) described the range of normal radiographic appearances of the breast as a function of age and menstrual status [Gershon-Cohen and Strickler 1938]. At that time, they noted that "considerable improvement of the Roentgen method will be necessary before it can be regarded as a superseding diagnostic aid in the early stages of breast pathology".

In 1951, an early version of the mammogram was proposed by Raúl *Alfredo* Leborgne (1907- 1986) [Leborgne 1951]. The idea was to compress the breast in order to enhance the image obtained from the x-rays. Leborgne reported finding radiographically visible microcalcifications in about 30% of breast cancers. Leborgne recommended the inclusion of Roentgen study in the diagnosis of mammary pathology.

In 1958, Gershon-Cohen and the pathologist Helen Ingleby (1887-1973) concluded that periodic mammograms of women older than 40 years would prove beneficial in reducing mortality from breast cancer [Gershon-Cohen and Ingleby 1958]. However, because their studies did not include controls, their work was largely ignored.

In 1960, Robert *Lee* Egan (1920-2001) adapted high-resolution industrial film to a mammographic technique [Egan 1960]. In a series of 1000 cases, a sensitivity of 97% was achieved, indicating the potential value of mammography both in the assessment of breast lesions and for screening asymptomatic women. This study contributed largely to move mammography into mainstream radiology.

During the 1960's-1970's, several prospective large-scale clinical trials were performed in an effort to determine the efficacy of screening mammography. The first of these (called "HIP study") was conducted on more than 60,000 women between the ages 40 and 64, from 1963 to 1967. The study found a one-third reduction in mortality from breast cancer at seven years' follow – up [Strax *et al.* 1973]. Another important study (called "BCDDP study") examined 280,000 women aged 35 to 74 years between 1973 and 1975

[Report of the working group to review the National Cancer Institute–American Cancer Society Breast Cancer Detection Demonstration Project. 1979; Smart *et al.* 1997]. These women were recruited to 29 locations and screened annually for 5 years with two-view mammography and clinical breast examination. BCDDP provided evidence that periodic mammography allowed detection of early malignant and even premalignant changes that were not recognized by women or their physicians during physical examination. This was confirmed by many subsequent randomized trials.

Before 1969, many "general-purpose" X-ray units were used that were not dedicated to mammography. These X-ray units had tungsten target tubes that were designed originally for medical imaging procedures, such as chest radiography. Some of these units had compression devices that were home made; therefore, breast compression was less than optimal by today's standards. Moreover, direct exposure (industrial type) X-ray films were being used, which often required long exposure times (causing blur by motion) and which resulted in high radiation exposure. Charles-*Marie* Gros (1910-1984), a physicist and physician at the University of Strasbourg, using a phantom, experimented with crystallographic X-ray tubes having different anode materials and filters. In 1969, based on the observations of Gros and colleagues, the first of series of dedicated mammographic X-ray units – the CGR ("Compagnie Générale de Radiologie") Sénographe (French for "picture of the breast") was commercialized. It used a molybdenum tube instead of a tungsten tube, allowing the delivery of a much lower level of radiation. It also offered images with greater contrast, improving the ability to see fine tissue variations. The built-in compression device narrowed the scatter range of the radiation; reduced shadowing caused by involuntary motion, and resulted in a clearer diagnostic image. Between 1969 and 1973, more than 1000 sénographes were installed.

In 1972, the first screen-film combination designed for mammography was introduced. With this single-screen, single-emulsion combination, radiation dose was reduced 10 to 20 times compared to direct exposure films. Most single-screen, single-emulsion film combinations commonly used today have higher film contrast and require significantly lower radiation exposure than those used a few years ago.

In the 1970's, as mammography was used to screen hundreds of thousands of women for breast cancer, the recourse to this modality was criticized, notably by John *Christian* Bailar III (b. 1932), a biostatistician and deputy associated director of NCI's cancer control program [Bailar 1976]. A political furor followed and, as the Bailar's warnings were widely publicized, the demand for mammography spectacularly declined. The debate centered on the dose of radiation used and its routine use in younger women. Today, technical improvements have significantly reduced the dose of radiation received during mammography, but routine mammograms for women under 50 are not widely supported. A schism between those who favored and opposed screening mammography still exists.

In 1997, diffraction enhanced X-ray imaging (DEI), a modification of the current practice of mammography, was introduced [Chapman *et al.* 1997]. In DEI, a silicon crystal is placed between the breast and the X-ray film or digital detector where the image is recorded. The crystal diffracts a particular wavelength of X-ray producing two images, based on absorption and refraction properties, respectively. The integration of these two images may provide more detail in the tissue. First reports on use of DEI with breast cancer specimens were done in 2000 [Pisano *et al.* 2000]. However, DEI is still in early stages of development and is not ready for clinical testing in 2010.

Computer-aided detection (CAD) systems for mammography became commercially available in 1998. Such systems have been approved by the FDA. They help increase the sensitivity for detecting small lesions and calcifications in the breast.

In 2000, the first full field digital mammography system approved by FDA, the Senographe 2000D, was introduced. The principle is similar to screen-film mammography except X-rays are recorded in digital format instead of on X-ray film. A main advantage of digital mammography compared to screen-film mammography is that the image acquisition, image display, and storage are decoupled. Digital mammography could be a better imaging tool and more accurate than conventional film mammography in 1) women under the age of 50 years; 2) women who are premenopausal or perimenopausal of age; and 3) women with radiographically dense breasts [Pisano *et al.* 2005].

While the primary benefit of digital mammography is a more reliable and efficient image management, an additional benefit is the ability to develop new clinical applications with the potential to improve breast cancer detection that were not possible with standard-film mammography, such as digital breast tomosynthesis (DBT) and contrast-enhanced digital mammography (CEM or CEDM). Introduced in the early 2000's, DBT is based on the acquisition of a three-dimensional volume of thin-section data (reviewed in [Park *et al.* 2007]). Images are reconstructed in conventional orientations by using reconstruction algorithms similar to those used in computed tomography (CT). This technique may improve the specificity of mammography with improved lesion margin visibility and may improve early breast cancer detection, especially in women with radiographically dense breasts, by avoiding the limitation of standard mammography, which attempts to project the three-dimensional anatomical information of the breast into a two-dimensional image [Niklason *et al.* 1997]. Currently, most mammograms are still performed on analog systems. CEM/CEDM, also introduced in the early 2000's is still in clinical trials. It has the potential to detect early stage breast malignancies by detecting signs of angiogenesis (increased formation of blood vessels). It uses an iodinated contrast agent (commonly used in CT imaging, such as Isovue or Omnipaque) injected into a vein, usually in the arm, in conjunction with a mammography examination. The images may highlight immature blood vessel development that often accompanies malignant growth [Dromain *et al.* 2009].

While breast self-examination and clinical breast examination remain the most obvious methods to discover breast problems, mammography was the most important advance made in the 20th century in the clinical detection of breast cancer. At present, mammography is still the gold standard for screening of the general population.

Magnetic Resonance Imaging (MRI)

Raymond *Vahan* Damadian (b. 1936) is credited of being the first to report, in 1971, that tumors and normal tissue could be distinguished *in vitro* by nuclear magnetic resonance (NMR) [Damadian 1971]. This produced a strong impetus for the use of NMR in medicine.

The NMR-based magnetic resonance imaging (MRI) was developed in 1973 by Paul *Christian* Lauterbur (1929-2007) and Peter Mansfield (b. 1933). Both received the Nobel Prize of Medicine in 2003. MRI imaging is based on the different signals obtained from different tissue types that are subjected to a high magnetic field (see notably [Lauterbur 1989]). Thus, MRI does not use ionizing radiations.

In the early 1980's, *in vivo* MR images of the breast were obtained by various investigators, but they failed to reach clinical value, notably due to poor spatial resolution. Starting from 1985, MR image quality was improved to a point that first criteria for benign and malignant breast lesions could be developed.

In 1986,contrast-enhanced MRI of the breast was introduced, with the complex gadolinium (Gd)-diethylenetriaminepentaacetic acid (DTPA) (also known as gadopentetate dimeglumine) as contrasting agent (see for instance

[Revel *et al.* 1986]). This substantially increased the information content of MR images.

In 1991, MRI was approved by FDA for use as a supplemental tool to mammography to help diagnose breast cancer. It may be used when screening mammograms demonstrate a questionable finding (other frequent alternatives are ultrasonography or biopsy). The addition of annual contrast-enhanced MRI of the breast to mammography, in the context of high risk screening, has revealed a significant reduction in breast cancer mortality for women aged 30 years or older who are known or likely to have inherited a strong predisposition to breast cancer [Warner 2008].

MRI is an excellent tool for imaging augmented breasts, including both the breast implant itself and the breast tissue surrounding the implant (abnormalities or signs of breast cancer can sometimes be obscured by the implant on a mammogram). In fact, contrast-enhanced MRI is currently considered to be the most sensitive imaging technique for breast cancer detection. However, MR imaging is limited by its high cost and the limited access.

In 1998, the first description of computer-aided detection (CAD) use in MRI was made [Gilhuijs *et al.* 1998]. CAD systems allow the radiologist to view up to 2000 images at one time. After the injection of contrast material and dynamic imaging, these systems color code the enhancement kinetics of various tissue areas of the breast. CAD systems help analyze enhancement patterns of tumor angiogenesis of invasive tumors versus normal fibroglandular tissue.

Of note, whole body MRI has been and is still used to detect skeletal metastases of breast cancer.

MRI Spectroscopy (or MRS)

Magnetic resonance spectroscopy (MRS) of intact biological tissues was first reported in 1973, in a study examining intact red blood cells [Moon and Richards 1973]. Still in the 1970's, MRS began to be applied to breast tumors. In MRI, the signal comes from protons mainly in water and lipids. In MRS, proton signals originate from hydrogen atoms attached to various metabolites of interest. In breast cancer, MRS is generally used to detect the increased content of "composite choline" (free choline, phosphocholine and glycerophosphocholine). Indeed, since the late 1990's, most reports in the literature have confirmed that there is increased "composite choline" metabolites in malignant lesions and this allows to differentiate between benign and malignant lesions (see notably [Tse *et al.* 2007]).

Ultrasonography

Ultrasonography (US) is an imaging technique in which high-frequency sound waves are reflected from tissues and internal organs.

In 1951, John *Julian Cuttance* Wild (1914-2009) and engineer Donald Neal could determine the acoustic characteristics of 2 breast tumors, 1 benign and 1 malignant, in the intact, *in vivo* breast with linear amplitude (A)-mode ultrasound transducer. They demonstrated qualitative differences between these tumors [Wild and Neal 1951] A-mode is the simplest type of ultrasound in which a single transducer scans a line through the body with the echoes plotted on screen as a function of depth.

In 1953, Wild and engineer John *Mitchell* Reid (born 1926) used a linear brightness (B)-mode US instrument to produce real-time images of a 7mm *in situ* cancer in an inflamed nipple (reported one year later: [Wild and Reid 1954]). Still in 1953, breast cysts were routinely diagnosed. In B-mode ultrasound, which is the most common use, a linear array of transducers simultaneously scans a plane through the body that can be viewed as a two-dimensional grey-scale image on screen.

By 1956, Wild and Reid had examined 117 cases of breast pathology with their linear real-time B-mode instrument. Data showed very promising results for pre-operative diagnosis. Malignant infiltration of tissues surrounding breast tumors could be resolved. Tumors as small as 1 mm were seen in the nipple.

B-mode scanning ultrasonography was approved by FDA in 1977 as an adjunct to mammography to evaluate suspicious areas on a mammogram, increasing the accuracy of the combined technologies.

In 1977, "conventional" Doppler ultrasound was first used for the benign-malignant differentiation of breast tumors [Wells *et al.* 1977]. As its name implies, this technique is based on the Doppler Effect, first described mathematically by the physicist Christian *Johann* Doppler (1803-1853). In breast cancer diagnostics, the moving objects measured by "Doppler effect" are blood cells and Doppler capability combined with B-mode US scanning may produce images of blood vessels from which blood flow can be directly measured.

The first automated ultrasound scanners were developed in the early 1980's.

Starting from 1990, Color Doppler ultrasound (CD-US) was used to study breast lesions [Adler et al. 1990]. Through the use of colors (red and blue) superimposed on a 2D gray scale image, CD-US may visualize the presence, direction and velocity of flowing blood in a wide range of flow conditions. CD-US is not as precise as conventional Doppler and is best used to scan a larger area and then use conventional Doppler for detailed analysis at a site of potential flow abnormality (for a review on CD-US, see [Athanasiou et al. 2009]).

In 1997 were published the first studies using Power Doppler ultrasound (PD-US) [Raza et al. 1997; Birdwell et al. 1997]. In PD-US, the power of the returning Doppler signal is measured, rather than the Doppler frequency shift, and it gives an estimation of the volume of moving blood rather than its velocity. A larger number of moving red cells gives a stronger Doppler signal than a smaller number, thus providing information on the volume of moving blood in the region of interest. As compared to CD-US, PD-US demonstrates the vascularity of tissues in more detail. It notably allows a better detection of small vessels, but is much more sensible to flow artifacts. As CD-US, PD-US is currently not widely used in clinical practice (for a review on PD-US, see [Athanasiou et al. 2009]).

Starting from mid-1990's, contrast-enhanced ultrasound (CE-US) was introduced (see notably [Kedar et al. 1996]). CE-US was mainly developed from 2000 [Chaudhari et al. 2000]. Ultrasound specific intravenous contrast agents typically consist of an encapsulating shell material (albumin, phospholipid or polymer) surrounding air or a fluorocarbon gas. These particles are relatively stable in the bloodstream and highly reflective of ultrasound at typical frequencies used in medical imaging. In general, the degree of increased echogenicity in a breast lesion will depend on the relative perfusion of the lesion compared to the parenchyma (thus yielding information similar to a contrast enhanced breast MRI).

In 1999, the first description of computer-aided detection (CAD) use in ultrasonography was made [Sawaki et al. 1999]. CAD US is still in clinical evaluation and certain preliminary studies have shown that it could improve the sensitivity and specificity of US [Athanasiou et al. 2009].

Three-dimensional (3D) US was introduced in breast imaging in the late 1990's (see notably [Carson et al. 1997]). It has the capacity to demonstrate lesion margins and topography, thereby helping differentiate benign from malignant masses. 3D-US offers a better appreciation of tumor volume, indispensable for monitoring patients under neo-adjuvant therapy. It can also help determine the need for biopsy and help facilitate needle localization and guidance during biopsy [Athanasiou *et al.* 2009]. 3D-Doppler US may be used to analyze the highly disorganized, tortuous and dilated blood vessels in a tumor vasculature as an adjunct parameter to help to improve the specificity of a diagnosis [Chang *et al.* 2007].

Tissue harmonic imaging (THI) of breast tumors was introduced in the early 2000's. When an ultrasound wave is transmitted into the body, reflected sound waves are produced at integral multiples of the transmission frequency, referred to as harmonics. Conventional B-mode US produces an image that represents the amplitude of reflected sound at the transmission frequency, or first harmonic. THI produces an image that represents the amplitude of higher order harmonics. Clinically, THI has proven very useful when scanning cystic breast lesions. The reduction of the "speckle artifact" which makes many cysts appear complicated has greatly helped with lesion characterization [Szopinski *et al.* 2003]. THI also has less penetration than images obtained with conventional sonography and it may therefore be necessary to use conventional ultrasound in order to fully visualize the deeper tissues in patients with large breasts [Athanasiou *et al.* 2009].

Compound Imaging (or compound US) of breast tumors was also introduced in the early 2000's. In conventional B-mode US, the image is constructed line-by-line at a constant angle of insonation. In compound US, the image is obtained by combining data from multiple different angles [Jespersen *et al.* 1998; Huber *et al.* 2002]. This can result in reduced image artifacts and improved image contrast, which notably ameliorates the detection of microcalcifications. Similar to THI images, specular echoes in simple cysts are reduced and normal breast ligaments, capsules and spiculations around masses are better seen. By providing a better definition of lesion lateral margins, it increases the conspicuity of small, subtle lesions [Athanasiou *et al.* 2009].

Thermoacoustic tomography (TAT) and photoacoustic tomography (PAT, also known as optoacoustic tomography -OAT-), introduced in the early 2000's, are based on the measurement of ultrasonic waves induced by electromagnetic radiation in the radiofrequency or microwave bands (for TAT) or visible or near infrared light (for PAT/OAT) (see for instance [Ermilov *et al.* 2009]). These non-invasive and non-ionizing imaging modalities can reveal dielectric or optical properties of tissues that are closely related to the physiological and pathological status of the tissues. They potentially provide high imaging contrast based on a tissue's rate of absorption of electromagnetic radiation [Ku *et al.* 2005]. Devices integrating the two imaging modalities into one system, making it easier to get an image at the same time, have been described [Pramanik *et al.* 2008]. Today, US is still the most important adjunctive imaging modality available for breast cancer diagnosis. It may distinguish between solid tumors and fluid-filled cysts with a near 100% accuracy [Coll 2008]. US is more sensitive than mammography for detecting abnormalities in dense breasts, hence it is more valuable in women younger than 35 in ages [Cheng *et al.* 2010]. It is also quite useful in conducting image-guided biopsy. One important reason for which ultrasonography is not currently used for routine breast cancer screening is that it does not consistently detect certain early signs of cancer such as microcalcifications, which are deposits of calcium in the breast that cannot be felt but can be seen on a conventional mammogram, and are the most common indicator of ductal carcinoma*in situ*. The role of ultrasound in breast tumor imaging has greatly expanded over the last ten years.

Optical Imaging

1) Transillumination – Diaphanography - Lightscanning

Optical imaging of breast cancers was first proposed in 1929, when Max Cutler (1899-1984) investigated the transmission of continuous wave visible light through the breast ("transillumination") to access masses [Cutler 1929]. However, the light intensity required caused overheating of the patient's skin. Moreover, no absorption quantification or high-resolution architectural information was available. Although cancerous lesions with increased vascularization were detected, certain other benign formations with increased hemoglobin content also yielded absorption contrast. Repeated attempts to improve the technique were un-successful, and it was temporarily abandoned in the 1940s (reviewed in [Ntziachristos and Chance 2001]).In the early 1970's, Cutler's work stimulated a more refined technique by Charles-*Marie* Gros (1910-1984) and his colleagues, which they termed "diaphanography" [Gros *et al.* 1972]. They used "cold" (visible or near-infrared) light that could penetrate even dense breast tissue and obtained an image of the transilluminated breast. Originally, these "images" were perceived by the physician's eye alone. Substantial improvements were made in the following decade, including the use of video cameras as detectors.Diaphanography was modified in 1982 [Carlsen 1982] by eliminating all light wavelengths except for visible red and near infrared, and combining transillumination with an electronic system that analyzed light over a wide spectrum, allowed real-time live viewing and stored the data for interpretation and retrieval. The process was called "lightscanning". However, the basic limitations that Max Cutler encountered almost 50 years ago, regarding differentiating between malignant and benign lesions, were not significantly improved by the use of better recording media. Furthermore, reports on the sensitivity of the method varied significantly, but several studies found that light scanning was inferior to traditional methods of breast imaging; the probability of detection was low for small cancers and the probability of false alarm was almost three times as high as that of other breast imaging methods.

2) Diffuse Optical Tomography (DOT)

Introduced in the late 1990's, DOT imaging employs diffuse light that propagates through tissue, at multiple projections, to yield three-dimensional quantified tomographic images of the internal optical properties of organs. Depending on the technology employed, DOT can yield quantified, three-dimensional maps of absorption, scattering, vascularization, oxygenation, and contrast agent uptake in either fluorescence or absorption mode. In comparison with transillumination, the technique offers superior quantification accuracy, independent determination of absorption, scattering and fluorescence lifetime and yield, three-dimensional imaging capability, and lesion size determination. DOT has recently been applied to clinical imaging of the breast, and prototype breast optical tomographic systems able to discriminate malignant from benign breast tissue in a reproducible qualitative and quantitative manner have been developed (see for instance [van de Ven *et al.* 2009]). However, because photons undergo multiple random scattering events as they propagate through highly-scattering tissue such as breast, DOT is incapable to detect small early-stage tumors or to resolve features at the cellular level.

3) Optical Coherence Tomography (OCT)

Introduced in the early 2000's, OCT is a high-resolution imaging technology that for larger and undifferentiated cells can perform cellular-level imaging at the expense of imaging depth. OCT performs optical ranging in tissue and is analogous to ultrasound except reflections of near-infrared light are detected rather than sound. While depth of imaging is limited to only a few millimeters in highly-scattering tissues, imaging resolutions less than 1micron have been demonstrated with OCT. With these high resolutions, OCT performs an 'optical biopsy', capturing images that approach the resolution and represent the architectural morphology commonly found in histology [Boppart *et al.* 2004].

4) Optoacoustic Tomography

Introduced in the early 2000's, but still largely experimental (see Ultrasound, in the "OAT" section)

Thermography

In 1956-1957, Canadian physician Raymond *Newton* Lawson (d.1996) introduced thermography (also called thermometry, thermology or, more recently, thermal imaging or infrared imaging) for breast cancer [Lawson 1957]. Thermography, which has been available since the 1960s, is based on the principle that the temperature in both pre-cancerous tissue and the area surrounding a developing breast cancer is almost always higher than in the normal breast. Since pre-cancerous and cancerous masses are highly metabolic tissues, they need an abundant supply of nutrients to maintain their growth. In order to do this they increase circulation to their cells by sending out chemicals to keep existing blood vessels open, recruit dormant vessels, and create new ones (neoangiogenesis). This process results in an increase in regional surface temperatures of the breast. Thermometry uses a thermal scanner to detect thermal emissions.

Through the 1960s and 1970s, thermography was generally well accepted and intensively studied. It was approved by the FDA in 1982 as a supplement to mammography in helping to detect breast cancer. However, due to a series of deceiving results, as compared to mammography (see for instance [Egan *et al.* 1977]), thermometry was progressively abandoned as a routine screening modality after the 1970s. Indeed, deep breast lesions often do not produce measurable changes, and many physiological conditions can cause changes in heat distribution, making of thermography a relatively non-specific test. Thus, though thermography was FDA approved, the modality has not gained wide acceptance in the medical community as a necessary or effective tool in breast cancer detection.

Computed Tomography (CT), Positron Emission Tomography (PET), Positron Emission Mammography (PEM), PET/CT

Computed Tomography (CT)

Although tomography (from the Greek *tomos* (slice)) was initially developed in the 1930's by Italian radiologist Alessandro Vallebona (1899-1987), the first computed tomography (CT) scan was created in 1971 by British electronics engineer Godfrey *Newbold* Hounsfield (1919-2004). In 1979, Hounsfield and South African nuclear physicist Allan *McLeod* Cormack (1924-1998) shared the Nobel Prize in physiology or medicine for the development of CT.CT uses X-rays and computer-assisted analysis to generate a three-dimensional image from flat (two-dimensional) X-ray pictures, one slice at a time. First results on the clinical value of CT in breast cancer were published in the late 1970's. Since, clinical trials have given contradictory results and the current opinion is that CT alone is inappropriate at least for screening purposes.In the future, however, CT could be used in association with PET (see below) and with SPECT (SPECT/CT, see below).

Positron Emission Tomography (PET)

The first human positron emission tomography (PET) scan was built in 1975 by Michael *Edward* Phelps (b. 1939) and Edward *Joseph* Hoffman (1942-2004). PET analysis is an imaging modality (scintigraphy) based on the detection of radiation emitted by a radiotracer, traditionally [F-18]-fluorodeoxyglucose (FDG). FDG frequently concentrates in malignant cells at a higher rate than in normal tissues.A PET tracer emits positrons which annihilate with electrons up to a few millimeters away, causing two gamma photons to be emitted and detected.As compared to MRI and CT, PET has the ability to inform about the biological activity of the area of interest as opposed to just its anatomic appearance. This allows for discrimination between objects that are non-living such as a scar from a growing group of cells such as those in a tumor.

First results on the clinical value of PET in breast cancer were published in the late 1980's (see notably [Minn and Soini 1989]). Although the sensitivity of whole-body PET is not very high, it is quite specific for the detection of metastatic disease.This has made the technology useful in breast cancer patients with either an advanced or recurrent disease. PET is also used for monitoring response to therapy. Indeed, anatomic methods require shrinkage of the tumor, and MRI has been shown to be quite accurate after 3–4 cycles (about 4 months) of treatment [Abraham*et al.* 1996]. Response to treatment can be seen by FDG-PET within 8 days [Wahl *et al.* 1993], long before the tumor shrinks. Recently, PET has been associated with mammography (PEM, see below). In the future, PET could also be used in association with CT (see PET/CT below). The medical necessity of PET scanning for oncologic applications depends, in part, on what imaging techniques are used either before or after PET scanning. PET scanning is typically considered after other techniques, such as computed tomography (CT), magnetic resonance imaging (MRI), or ultrasonography, provide inconclusive or discordant results.

Positron Emission Mammography (PEM)

The first feasibility study on positron emission mammography (PEM) technology was published in 1994 [Thompson *et al.* 1994]. First results on the clinical value of PEM in breast cancer were published in the early 2000's (see notably [Levine *et al.* 2003]).Positron emission mammography (PEM) technology uses two planar detectors integrated into a conventional mammography system that enables the coregistration of a mammographic and emission FDG image. As compared to whole-body PET scanners, the PEM exam captures localized images of the breast, producing very sharp, detailed images of breast lesions – as small as 1.5 – 2mm. PEM promises enhanced detection of ductal carcinoma*in situ* (DCIS), even when not associated with microcalcifications, of small tumors that have not been imaged with MRI, mammography or US, and may also help tailor breast-surgical procedures [Tafra 2007]. Further study of this issue is warranted.

PET/CT

PET/CT combines the functional information and metabolic sensitivity provided by PET with the anatomic data and the temporal and spatial resolution offered by CT into one scanner [Beyer *et al.* 2002; Zangheri *et al.* 2004].While the results from a majority of the published studies on PET/CT fusion are preliminary and have focused on assessing technical feasibility and potential clinical applications, it can already be stated that this diagnostic tool improves upon imaging by using PET alone, because it synthesizes both structural and metabolic information. Early studies suggest that this additional information may help alter treatment decisions. From a practical perspective, there is now a movement toward utilizing PET/CT imaging for any oncologic indication where PET scanning would be indicated, i.e., for the diagnosis, staging, and monitoring of treatment for a number of different malignancies. Specifically, several small studies have suggested that PET/CT fusion has improved diagnostic ability over PET alone in lung cancer, lymphoma, malignant melanoma, and a variety of gastrointestinal, gynecological and head and neck malignancies. PET/CT fusion may be considered medically necessary for any oncologic indication where PET scanning is considered medically necessary.

PET/CT has a role in detecting local disease recurrence and distant metastasis in breast cancer patients [Singh *et al.* 2008].

PET scans with or without PET/CT fusion are considered medically necessary for the following oncologic indications:

1) to evaluate the presence of metastases in high risk patients where standard imaging is inconclusive;
2) when progressive disease is suspected on the basis of rising markers and standard imaging is inconclusive;
3) for monitoring tumor response in those patients in whom PET scans have been established as the only technique to follow disease.

Scintigraphy, Single Photon Emission Computed Tomography (SPECT), SPECT/CT, Scintimammography, BSGI

Scintigraphy

The first attempts to visualize breast tumors with radioactive compounds were made in the late 1960's and early 1970's (see for instance [Cancroft and Goldsmith 1973]). The tracer used in scintigraphy emits gamma (γ) radiation that is measured directly by a γ-camera.

Scintigraphy has been used to detect lymph node metastases (lymphoscintigraphy), bone metastases (bone scintigraphy, which is recommended as the first imaging study in patients who are asymptomatic) and as adjunct to mammography for the diagnosis of breast cancer (mammoscintigraphy or scintimammography).

Introduced in clinical imaging in the early 1990's, technetium (99mTc) sestamibi (MIBI) is still the most used radiotracer in scintigraphy.

Single Photon Emission Computed Tomography (SPECT)

SPECT is a tomographic version of conventional (planar) scintigraphy. It uses the same radiopharmaceuticals but provides 3D images of the concentration of the radiotracer, through the use of a rotating camera (tomography).

It results better contrast and resolution. SPECT is similar to PET in its use of radioactive tracer material and detection of γ-rays. PET provides higher resolution images than SPECT (which has about 1 cm resolution).

SPECT scans, however, are significantly less expensive than PET scans, in part because they are able to use longer-lived more easily-obtained radioisotopes than PET. SPECT is used notably for bone scan using bisphosphonates labelled with 99mTc, or tumor scan using (99mTc)MIBI. To date, SPECT is considered investigational and not medically necessary for breast cancer scintigraphy.

Single Photon Emission Computed Tomography/Computed Tomography (SPECT/CT)

SPECT/CT merges the information provided by SPECT with the anatomical details obtained from CT.It was introduced in the early 2000's [Keydar et al. 2003] and is used in breast cancer patients since 2007, mainly for lymphatic (sentinel node) mapping, as it appears better than conventional imaging for the confirmation of the exact anatomic location of a sentinel node [van der Ploeg et al. 2007]. To date, SPECT/CT is considered investigational and not medically necessary for breast cancer imaging.

Scintimammography and BSGI

Introduced in the mid-2000s, breast-specific gamma (γ) imaging (BSGI) is a scintimammography, thus a scintigraphy restricted to breast, in which (99mTc)MIBI-emitted γ-rays are detected by a high-resolution breast-optimized γ-camera. BSGI is most commonly used for patients who have equivocal mammography or ultrasound findings. It is also used to help determine the extent of breast cancer involvement and to help clarify lymph-node involvement. Larger, multicenter studies are needed to validate the potential of BSGI as an adjunct screening or diagnostic modality and to further identify the subset of patients for whom this technology will improve net health outcomes and contribute to clinical management.

Elastography

The theoretical and practical basis for elastography was given in 1999 [Ophir *et al.* 1999]. In elastography, the stiffness of breast tissues in response to a mechanical stimulus are measured from point to point within the breast by ultrasonography or MRI. These measurements are mapped into images, often called "elastograms".

Elastic properties of tissues can be determined by ultrasound or MRI obtained before and after application of small deformations or by monitoring the propagation of mechanical (infrasonic) waves. Ultrasonic and magnetic resonance elastography have the potential to distinguish breast abnormalities, such as malignant tumors, from normal tissue, benign processes, and scars. Since, in general, elastography can be done noninvasively to form images for subjective and quantitative evaluation, these methods are under active evaluation. Elastic properties are not directly measured, however, and must be inferred (mathematically) by one of numerous technical strategies used to model and display the images.

No extensive clinical trials of elastography in breast cancer have yet been reported, but some feasibility demonstrations have been completed, so such trials are anticipated [Plewes *et al.* 2000; Sinkus *et al.* 2000]. However, assessment of elastography could be hampered by a lack of standardization with regard to which elastic parameters should be measured and by a lack of published characterization of normal tissue.

Electrical Impedance Tomography

Introduced in the early 2000s, electrical impedance scanning of the breast involves the transmission of continuous electricity into the body using either an electrical patch attached to the arm or a hand held cylinder. The electrical current travels through the breast where it is then measured at skin level by a probe placed on the breast. The basic principle of this technique is that cancerous tissue conducts electricity differently than normal tissue. As the probe is placed over various locations on the breast, the electrical impedance encountered by the probe, changes if cancerous tissue is encountered. This change in impedance, corresponding to the location of a cancerous lesion, is then represented as a bright white spot on the computerized image. Electrical impedance scanning of the breast is considered investigational/not medically necessary for all indications. (for a review, see [Fass 2008])

References

Abraham DC, Jones RC, Jones SE, Cheek JH, Peters GN, Knox SM, Grant MD, Hampe DW, Savino DA, Harms SE. Evaluation of neoadjuvant chemotherapeutic response of locally advanced breast cancer by magnetic resonance imaging. *Cancer.* 1996 Jul 1;78(1):91-100.

Adler DD, Carson PL, Rubin JM, Quinn-Reid D. Doppler ultrasound color flow imaging in the study of breast cancer: preliminary findings. Ultrasound Med Biol. 1990;16(6):553-9; Cosgrove DO, Bamber JC, Davey JB, McKinna JA, Sinnett HD. Color Doppler signals from breast tumors. Work in progress. *Radiology.* 1990 Jul;176(1):175-80.

Athanasiou A, Tardivon A, Ollivier L, Thibault F, El Khoury C, Neuenschwander S. How to optimize breast ultrasound. *Eur. J. Radiol.* 2009 Jan;69(1):6-13.

Bailar JC 3rd. Mammography: A Contrary View. *Ann. Intern.Med.* 1976 Jan;84(1):77-84.

Beyer T, Townsend DW, Blodgett TM. Dual-modality PET/CT tomography for clinical oncology. *Q J Nucl. Med.* 2002 Mar;46(1):24-34.

Birdwell RL, Ikeda DM, Jeffrey SS, Jeffrey RB Jr. Preliminary experience with power Doppler imaging of solid breast masses. *AJR Am. J.Roentgenol.* 1997 Sep;169(3):703-7.

Boppart SA, Luo W, Marks DL, Singletary KW. Optical coherence tomography: feasibility for basic research and image-guided surgery of breast cancer. *Breast Cancer Res. Treat.* 2004 Mar;84(2):85-97.

Cancroft ET, Goldsmith SJ. 99m Tc-pertechnetate scintigraphy as an aid in the diagnosis of breast masses. *Radiology.* 1973 Feb;106(2):441-4.

Carlsen E. Transillumination light scanning. *Diagn. Imaging.* 1982;4:28-34.

Carson PL, Moskalik AP, Govil A, Roubidoux MA, Fowlkes JB, Normolle D, Adler DD, Rubin JM, Helvie M. The 3D and 2D color flow display of breast masses. *Ultrasound Med. Biol.* 1997;23(6):837-49.

Chang RF, Huang SF, Moon WK, et al. Solid breast masses: neural network analysis of vascular features at three-dimensional power Doppler US for benign or malignant classification. *Radiology.* 2007;243(1):56-62.

Chapman D, Thomlinson W, Johnston RE, Washburn D, Pisano E, Gmür N, Zhong Z, Menk R, Arfelli F, Sayers D. Diffraction enhanced x-ray imaging. *Phys. Med. Biol.* 1997 Nov;42(11):2015-25.

Chaudhari MH, Forsberg F, Voodarla A, Saikali FN, Goonewardene S, Needleman L, Finkel GC, Goldberg BB. Breast tumor vascularity identified by contrast enhanced ultrasound and pathology: initial results. *Ultrasonics.* 2000 Mar;38(1-8):105-9.

Cheng HD, Shan J, Ju W, Guo Y, Zhang L. Automated breast cancer detection and classification using ultrasound images: A survey. *Patt Recog.* 2010; 43(1):299-317.

Coll D. Breast tumor imaging. *Cancer Treat Res.* 2008;143:515-46.

Cutler M. Transillumination as an aid in the diagnosis of breast lesions. *Surg.Gynecol. Obstet.* 1929; 48:721-9.

Damadian R. Tumor Detection by Nuclear Magnetic Resonance. *Science.* 1971 Mar 19;171(976):1151-3.

Dromain C, Balleyguier C, Adler G, Garbay JR, Delaloge S. Contrast-enhanced digital mammography. *Eur. J. Radiol.* 2009 Jan;69(1):34-42.

Egan RL. Experience with mammography in a tumour institute. Evaluation of 1000 studies. *Radiology.* 1960 Dec;75:894-900.

Egan RL, Goldstein GT, McSweeney MM. Conventional mammography, physical examination, thermography and xeroradiography in the detection of breast cancer. *Cancer.* 1977 May;39(5):1984-92.

Ermilov SA, Khamapirad T, Conjusteau A, Leonard MH, Lacewell R, Mehta K, Miller T, Oraevsky AA. Laser optoacoustic imaging system for detection of breast cancer. J Biomed Opt. 2009 Mar-Apr;14(2):024007

Fass L. Imaging and cancer: a review. *Mol. Oncol.* 2008 Aug;2(2):115-52.

Fray WW, Warren SL. Stereoscopic Röntgenography of the Breasts: An Aid in Establishing the Diagnosis of Mastitis and Carcinoma. *Ann. Surg.* 1932 Mar;95(3):425-32.

Gershon-Cohen J, Strickler A. Roentgenologic examination of the normal breast: its evaluation in demonstrating early neoplastic changes. *AJR* 1938; 40:189-201.

Gershon-Cohen J, Ingleby H. Roentgenography of unsuspected carcinoma of breast. *J. Am. Med. Assoc.* 1958 Feb 22;166(8):869–873.

Gilhuijs KG, Giger ML, Bick U. Computerized analysis of breast lesions in three dimensions using dynamic magnetic-resonance imaging. *Med. Phys.* 1998 Sep;25(9):1647-54.

Gros CM, Quenneville Y, Hummel YJ. Diaphanologie mammaire. *Radiol.Electrol. Med. Nucl.* 1972; 53:297-306.

Huber S, Wagner M, Medl M, Czembirek H. Real time spatial compound imaging in breast ultrasound. *Ultrason. Imaging.* 1998 Apr;20(2):81-102.

Jespersen SK, Wilhjelm JE, Sillesen H. Multiangle compound imaging. *Ultrason.Imaging* 1998; 20:81–102.

Kedar RP, Cosgrove D, McCready VR, Bamber JC, Carter ER. Microbubble contrast agent for color Doppler US: effect on breast masses. Work in progress. *Radiology.* 1996 Mar;198(3):679-86

Keydar Z, Israel O, Krausz Y. SPECT/CT in tumor imaging: technical aspects and clinical applications. *Semin. Nucl. Med.* 2003 Jul;33(3):205-18.

Ku G, Fornage BD, Jin X, Xu M, Hunt KK, Wang LV. Thermoacoustic and photoacoustic tomography of thick biological tissues toward breast imaging. *Technol. Cancer Res. Treat.* 2005 Oct;4(5):559-66.

Lauterbur PC. Image formation by induced local interactions. Examples employing nuclear magnetic resonance. Clin Orthop Relat Res. 1989 Jul;(244):3-6.

Lawson R. Thermography; a new tool in the investigation of breast lesions. *Can. Serv. Med. J.* 1957 Sep;8(8):517-24.

Leborgne R. Diagnosis of tumors of the breast by simple roentgenography; calcifications in carcinomas. *Am. J. Roentgenol. Radium. Ther.* 1951 Jan;65(1):1-11.

Levine EA, Freimanis RI, Perrier ND, Morton K, Lesko NM, Bergman S, Geisinger KR, Williams RC, Sharpe C, Zavarzin V, Weinberg IN, Stepanov PY, Beylin D, Lauckner K, Doss M, Lovelace J, Adler LP. Positron emission mammography: initial clinical results. *Ann. Surg. Oncol.* 2003 Jan-Feb;10(1):86-91.

Minn H, Soini I. [18F]fluorodeoxyglucose scintigraphy in diagnosis and follow up of treatment in advanced breast cancer. *Eur. J. Nucl. Med. 1989*; 15(2):61-6.

Moon RB, Richards JH. Determination of intracellular pH by 31P magnetic resonance. *J. Biol. Chem.* 1973 Oct 25;248(20):7276-8.

Niklason LT, Christian BT, Niklason LE, Kopans DB, Castleberry DE, Opsahl-Ong BH, Landberg CE, Slanetz PJ, Giardino AA, Moore R, Albagli D, DeJule MC, Fitzgerald PF, Fobare DF, Giambattista BW, Kwasnick RF, Liu J, Lubowski SJ, Possin GE, Richotte JF, Wei CY, Wirth RF. Digital tomosynthesis in breast imaging. *Radiology.* 1997 Nov;205(2):399-406.

Ntziachristos V, Chance B. Breast imaging technology: Probing physiology and molecular function using optical imaging - applications to breast cancer. *Breast Cancer Res.* 2001;3(1):41-6.

Ophir J, Alam SK, Garra B, Kallel F, Konofagou E, Krouskop T, Varghese T. Elastography: ultrasonic estimation and imaging of the elastic properties of tissues. *Proc. Inst. Mech. Eng* [H]. 1999;213(3):203-33.

Park JM, Franken EA Jr, Garg M, Fajardo LL, Niklason LT. Breast tomosynthesis: present considerations and future applications. *Radiographics.* 2007 Oct;27 Suppl 1:S231-40.

Pisano ED, Johnston RE, Chapman D, Geradts J, Iacocca MV, Livasy CA, Washburn DB, Sayers DE, Zhong Z, Kiss MZ, Thomlinson WC. Human breast cancer specimens: diffraction-enhanced imaging with histologic correlation--improved conspicuity of lesion detail compared with digital radiography. *Radiology.* 2000 Mar;214(3):895-901.

Pisano ED, Gatsonis C, Hendrick E, Yaffe M, Baum JK, Acharyya S, Conant EF, Fajardo LL, Bassett L, D'Orsi C, Jong R, Rebner M; Digital Mammographic Imaging Screening Trial (DMIST) Investigators Group. Diagnostic performance of digital versus film mammography for breast-cancer screening. *N. Engl. J. Med.* 2005 Oct 27;353(17):1773-83.

Plewes DB, Bishop J, Samani A, Sciarretta J. Visualization and quantification of breast cancer biomechanical properties with magnetic resonance elastography. *Phys. Med. Biol.* 2000 Jun;45(6):1591-610.

Pramanik M, Ku G, Li C, Wang LV. Design and evaluation of a novel breast cancer detection system combining both thermoacoustic (TA) and photoacoustic (PA) tomography. *Med. Phys.* 2008 Jun;35(6):2218-23.

Raza S, Baum JK. Solid breast lesions: evaluation with power Doppler US. *Radiology.* 1997 Apr;203(1):164-8.

Report of the working group to review the National Cancer Institute–American Cancer Society Breast Cancer Detection Demonstration Project. *J. Natl.Cancer Inst* 1979;62:639-709.

Revel D, Brasch RC, Paajanen H, Rosenau W, Grodd W, Engelstad B, Fox P, Winkelhake J. Gd-DTPA contrast enhancement and tissue differentiation in MR imaging of experimental breast carcinoma. *Radiology.* 1986 Feb;158(2):319-23.

Salomon A: Beitrage zur Pathologie und Klinik der Mammacarcinome. *Arch. Kein. Chir.* 1913;110:573–668.

Sawaki A, Shimamoto K, Satake H, Ishigaki T, Koyama S, Obata Y, Ikeda M. Breast ultrasonography: diagnostic efficacy of a computer-aided diagnostic system using fuzzy inference. *Radiat Med.* 1999 Jan-Feb;17(1):41-5.

Singh V, Saunders C, Wylie L, Bourke A. New diagnostic techniques for breast cancer detection. *Future Oncol.* 2008 Aug;4(4):501-13.

Sinkus R, Lorenzen J, Schrader D, Lorenzen M, Dargatz M, Holz D. High-resolution tensor MR elastography for breast tumour detection. *Phys. Med.Biol.* 2000 Jun;45(6):1649-64.

Smart CA, Byrne CA, Smith RA: Twenty-year follow-up of the breast cancers diagnosed during the Breast Cancer Detection Demonstration Project. *CACancer J. Clin.* 1997;47:134-149.

Strax P, Venet L, Shapiro S. Value of mammography in reduction of mortality from breast cancer in mass screening. *Am. J. Roentgenol. Radium. Ther. Nucl. Med.* 1973;117:686–9.

Szopinski KT, Pajk AM, Wysocki M, et al: Tissue harmonic imaging: utility in breast sonography. *J. Ultrasound Med* 22:479-487, 2003.

Tafra L. Positron Emission Tomography (PET) and Mammography (PEM) for breast cancer: importance to surgeons. *Ann. Surg. Oncol.* 2007 Jan;14(1):3-13.

Thompson CJ, Murthy K, Weinberg IN, Mako F. Feasibility study for positron emission mammography. *Med. Phys.* 1994 Apr;21(4):529-38.

Tse GM, Yeung DK, King AD, Cheung HS, Yang WT. In vivo proton magnetic resonance spectroscopy of breast lesions: an update. *Breast Cancer Res. Treat.* 2007 Sep;104(3):249-55.

van der Ploeg IM, Valdés Olmos RA, Nieweg OE, Rutgers EJ, Kroon BB, Hoefnagel CA. The additional value of SPECT/CT in lymphatic mapping in breast cancer and melanoma. *J. Nucl. Med.* 2007 Nov;48(11):1756-60.

van de Ven SM, Elias SG, Wiethoff AJ, van der Voort M, Nielsen T, Brendel B, Bontus C, Uhlemann F, Nachabe R, Harbers R, van Beek M, Bakker L, van der Mark MB, Luijten P, Mali WP. Diffuse optical tomography of the breast: preliminary findings of a new prototype and comparison with magnetic resonance imaging. *Eur. Radiol.* 2009 May;19(5):1108-13.

Wahl RL, Zasadny K, Helvie M, Hutchins GD, Weber B, Cody R. Metabolic monitoring of breast cancer chemohormonotherapy using positron emission tomography: initial evaluation. *J. Clin. Oncol.* 1993 Nov;11(11):2101-11.

Warner E. The role of magnetic resonance imaging in screening women at high risk of breast cancer. *Top Magn. Reson. Imaging* 2008;19:163–9.

Warren SL. Röntgenological study of the breast. *Am. J. Röntgen.* 1930;24:113

Wells PT, Halliwell M, Skidmore R, Webb AJ, Woodcock JP. Tumour detection by ultrasonic Doppler blood-flow signals. *Ultrasonics.* 1977 Sep;15(5):231-2.

Wild JJ, Neal D. Use of high-frequency ultrasonic waves for detecting changes of texture in living tissues. *Lancet.* 1951 Mar 24;1(6656):655-7.

Wild JJ, Reid JM.Echographic Visualization of Lesions of the Living Intact Human Breast. *Cancer Res.* 1954 May;14(4):277-82.

Zangheri B, Messa C, Picchio M, Gianolli L, Landoni C, Fazio F. PET/CT and breast cancer. *Eur. J. Nucl. Med. Mol. Imaging.* 2004 Jun;31 Suppl 1:S135-42.

Chapter 12

Twentieth Century and Beyond Breast Cancer Models

Abstract

During the 20th century, the elucidation of the causes and of the mechanisms of cancer initiation and progression has widely benefited from the introduction and intensive use of "cancer models". These include genetically well-characterized and genetically modified rodents, xenografts, cell lines (of which the three most used are MCF-7, T-47D and MDA-MB-231) and mammospheres. Models generally provided more reproducible experimental conditions and abundant tumor material for *in vitro* as well as *in vivo* research. In most cases, the relevance of these models has been shown.

Mouse Models

The first animal models widely used for breast cancer research were strains of mice. In 1916, Abbie Lathrop (1868-1918), a retired school teacher turned into a mouse breeder, and German-born American physician Leo Loeb (1869-1959) [Suntzeff 1960] used such models to show that oophorectomy prevented the development of mammary tumors [Lathrop and Loeb 1916]. Until her death, Lathrop interacted with biologists, including those from Harvard University, in such a way that many of the mouse strains used by scientists today originate from Lathrop's mice. American geneticist Clarence

Cook Little (1888-1971) took some of Lathrop's mice to establish the first "inbred" strains; mice bred to contain the same sets of genes [Shimkin 1975].

Strains of mice with a high incidence of spontaneous mammary tumors were intensively used as laboratory models. However, in 1936, the "Bittner milk factor", named after geneticist John *Joseph* Bittner (1904-1961), was discovered [Bittner 1936]. Subsequent studies indicated that a virus (a retrovirus later named "Mouse Mammary Tumor Virus", or MMTV) was able to transmit mammary carcinogenesis to subsequent generations through the mother's milk (for a review on MMTV, see [Callahan and Smith 2000]).

After Bittner's observations, and as the research community began to realize that breast cancer was not, in the vast majority of cases, a viral disease (see chapter 10), mouse models fell out of fashion, until the development of genetically engineered mice (GEM) and of breast cancer xenografts (see below). In the 21st century, mouse models are notably used to study the behavior (metastasis and response to drugs) of human breast cancer cells, using xenografts or cell lines (for recent reviews, see: [Man *et al.* 2007; Allred and Medina 2008]. Mice are not men, however, and some aspects of breast cancer, particularly steroid hormone dependence, are not well modeled in mice. For instance, initial tumor testing of tamoxifen in mice revealed that it was an estrogen in the mouse, while being mainly an antiestrogen in women. This pharmacologic peculiarity became important later with the recognition of selective estrogen receptor modulation [Jordan and Robinson 1987].

Rat Models

Various agents have been shown to induce mammary carcinogenesis in the rat, but premalignant stages of the disease have been best characterized in chemically-induced models, specifically those initiated by either 7,12 dimethylbenz[alpha]anthracene (DMBA) or 1-methyl-1-nitrosourea (MNU, also known as NMU or N-nitroso-N-methylurea) (for a review, see [Thompson and Singh 2000]).

In the late 1960's, the DMBA rat mammary carcinoma model, introduced by Canadian-born, American physician Charles *Brenton* Huggins (1901-1997) [Huggins *et al.* 1961], was extremely fashionable for research on the endocrinology of rat mammary carcinogenesis. Indeed, in contrast to most mammary tumors that arise in genetically engineered mice (GEM), which are hormone-independent, chemically-induced rat mammary tumors are generally hormone-dependent adenocarcinomas. It seems that the histogenesis of lesionsoccurring in chemically induced mammary carcinogenesis in the rat is similar to that observed in the human. However, the spectrum of lesions observed in the rat is limited, rat mammary tumors rarely metastasize [Russo and Russo 2000], and are regulated primarily by prolactin secreted by the pituitary gland in direct response to estrogen action [Lieberman *et al.* 1978].

Breast Cancer Cell (BCC) Lines

In 1958, and although some earlier attempts had been documented, the first stable, continuous culture of a human breast cancer cell (BCC) line, BT-20, was obtained by Etienne Yves Lasfargues (b. 1916) and Luciano Ozzello (b. 1926) from a multicentric, rapidly invading carcinoma [Lasfargues and Ozzello 1958]. Propagation of human BCCs in long term culture proved initially to be particularly difficult, as attempts to culture breast cancer cells from primary tumors have been largely unsuccessful.

In 1973, the estrogen receptor-positive MCF-7 cell line, which has become the most-used breast cancer cell line, was established [Soule *et al.* 1973; Levenson and Jordan 1997]. MCF-7 and most of the currently available BCC lines issued from metastatic tumors, mainly from pleural effusions. Effusions provide generally large numbers of dissociated, viable tumor cells with little or no contamination by fibroblasts and other tumor stoma cells [Lacroix and Leclercq 2004]. Another widely-used estrogen receptor-positive BCC line is T-47D [Keydar *et al.* 1979].

In 1974, the second most frequently-used BCC line, MDA-MB-231, was established [Cailleau *et al.* 1974]. Many of the currently used BCC lines were established in the 1970's. In 2004, MCF-7, T-47D, and MDA-MB-231, accounted for more than two-thirds of all abstracts reporting studies on mentioned BCC lines, as concluded from a Medline (http://www.ncbi.nlm.nih.gov/PubMed/)-based survey [Lacroix and Leclercq 2004]. Other BCC lines are used as they express interesting distinctive features. This is the case for BT-474 and SK-BR-3, which have an amplified *ERBB2* gene (encoding HER2/neu) at 17q11.2-q12 and overexpress HER2/neu. HS578T BCC originated from a carcinosarcoma, a rare form of breast cancer [Hackett et al. 1977]. HCC1937 is homozygous for the BRCA1 5382insC mutation and is derived from a germ-line BRCA1 mutation carrier [Tomlinson *et al.* 1998]. For additional information about these and other BCC lines, see [Lacroix and Leclercq 2004].

Of note, another cell line, MDA-MB-435, isolated in 1978 as "breast cancer cells" [Cailleau *et al.* 1978] and widely-used for about 30 years due to their high invasiveness in mouse models, have recently been requalified as "melanoma cells" [Lacroix 2008, Lacroix 2009], underlying the importance of checking the authenticity of cancer cell lines used in the laboratories.

BCC lines have been precious in investigating how proliferation, apoptosis and migration are deregulated during the progression of breast cancer. They are easily propagated, relatively tractable to genetic manipulation and under well-defined experimental conditions, generally yield reproducible and quantifiable results.

Moreover, many cell lines can be also grown in xenografts or in non-adherent mammospheres (see below) [Vargo-Gogola and Rosen 2007].

BCC lines are generally cultured on plastic, thus in bi-dimensional (2D) culture conditions. This results in the loss of structure and tissue function, as compared to breast tumors, in which cancer cells are embedded in a three-dimensional (3D) extracellular matrix. Since the early 2000's, attempts have been made to develop 3D culture methods for BCC. This has notably been pioneered by Mina *Jahan* Bissell (b. 1940) and colleagues (for a review, see [Weigelt and Bissell 2008])

Breast Cancer Xenografts

In 1974, the first breast cancer xenograft was described, as MX-1 (Mammary Xenograft-1), diagnosed histologically as an infiltrating duct cell carcinoma, was established in athymic nude mice in the National Cancer Institute and passaged by subcutaneous transplantation [Giovanella *et al.* 1974].

A few xenograft lines derived directly from primary cancers have been used in breast cancer studies; the most widely used xenografts in breast cancer have been those derived from established human breast cancer cell lines, such as MCF-7 or MDA-MB-231.

Rats and hamsters were also, but less frequently, used to receive xenografts. The ability to maintain and study breast tumors in an in vivo environment has proved to be a valuable tool in breast cancer research for several decades.

While xenografts are often obtained using injected BCC lines, breast cancer clinical isolates may also be used. However, transplantation efficiency of these primary breast cancer xenografts is generally poor.

Genetically Engineered Mice (GEM)

The first GEM were developed in the early 1980's (see notably [Stewart *et al.* 1984] and the review by [Leder and Stewart 1984]). They have contributed extensively to our understanding of genes, including tumor suppressor genes and oncogenes that are involved in the promotion and progression of breast cancer.

The first transgenes were made of putative oncogenes downstream of MMTV or "Whey Acidic Protein" (Wap) promoters. Advances in genetic engineering have allowed more precise control of the developmental timing of loss or gain of gene function, tissue selectivity and targeting of particular cell types in GEM.

Mammospheres

Nonadherent mammospheres were introduced in the mid-1990. They are spherical colonies formed by mammary epithelial cells when they are cultured on nonadherent surfaces in the presence of growth factors [Hurley *et al.* 1994].

In 2003, it was shown that nonadherent mammospheres were enriched in cells with functional characteristics of stem/progenitor cells [Dontu *et al.* 2003]. More recently, mammosphere culture has been used to identify and study potential breast cancer stem cells (see notably [Li *et al.* 2008; Grimshaw *et al.* 2008]).

Breast Cancer Stem Cells

Starting from the early 2000's, it has been suggested that breast tumors and BCC lines could contain tumor-initiating subpopulations ("breast cancer stem cells" or BCSC).

Due to their resistance to drugs and radiation, such cells could evade therapy and cause the tumors to re-grow. While these BCSC could be useful models to study resistances and develop new therapeutic approaches, improved methods and markers are needed to identify and characterize these cells within cell lines and tumors (for a review on BCSC, see [Charafe-Jauffret *et al.* 2009]).

References

Allred DC, Medina D. The relevance of mouse models to understanding the development and progression of human breast cancer. *J. Mammary GlandBiol. Neoplasia.* 2008 Sep;13(3):279-88.

Bittner JJ. Some possible effects of nursing on the mammary gland tumor incidence in mice. *Science.* 1936 Aug 14;84(2172):162.

Cailleau R, Young R, Olivé M, Reeves WJ Jr. Breast tumor cell lines from pleural effusions. *J. Natl. Cancer Inst.* 1974 Sep;53(3):661-74.

Cailleau R, Olivé M, Cruciger QV. Long-term human breast carcinoma cell lines of metastatic origin: preliminary characterization. In Vitro. 1978 Nov;14(11):911-5.

Callahan R, Smith GH. MMTV-induced mammary tumorigenesis: gene discovery, progression to malignancy and cellular pathways. *Oncogene.* 2000 Feb 21;19(8):992-1001.

Charafe-Jauffret E, Ginestier C, Birnbaum D. Breast cancer stem cells: tools and models to rely on. *BMC Cancer.* 2009 Jun 25;9:202.

Dontu G, Abdallah WM, Foley JM, Jackson KW, Clarke MF, Kawamura MJ, Wicha MS. In vitro propagation and transcriptional profiling of human mammary stem/progenitor cells. *Genes Dev.* 2003 May 15;17(10):1253-70.

Giovanella BC, Stehlin JS, Williams LJ: Heterotransplantation of human malignant tumors in "nude" thymusless mice. 11. Malignant tumors induced by injection of cell cultures derived from human solid tumors. *J. Natl. Cancer Inst.* 1974 Mar;52(3):921-30..

Grimshaw MJ, Cooper L, Papazisis K, Coleman JA, Bohnenkamp HR, Chiapero-Stanke L, Taylor-Papadimitriou J, Burchell JM. Mammosphere culture of metastatic breast cancer cells enriches for tumorigenic breast cancer cells. *Breast Cancer Res.* 2008;10(3):R52.

Hackett AJ, Smith HS, Springer EL, Owens RB, Nelson-Rees WA, Riggs JL, Gardner MB. Two syngeneic cell lines from human breast tissue: the aneuploid mammary epithelial (Hs578T) and the diploid myoepithelial (Hs578Bst) cell lines. *J. Natl. Cancer Inst.* 1977 Jun;58(6):1795-806.

Huggins C, Morii S, Grand LC. Mammary cancer induced by a single dose of polynuclear hydrocarbons: routes of administration. *Ann. Surg.* 1961 Dec;154(6)Suppl:315-8.

Hurley WL, Blatchford DR, Hendry KA, Wilde CJ. Extracellular matrix and mouse mammary cell function: comparison of substrata in culture. *In Vitro Cell Dev. Biol. Anim.* 1994 Aug;30A(8):529-38.

Jordan VC, Robinson SP. Species-specific pharmacology of antiestrogens: role of metabolism. *Fed. Proc.* 1987 Apr;46(5):1870-4.

Keydar I, Chen L, Karby S, Weiss FR, Delarea J, Radu M, Chaitcik S, Brenner HJ. Establishment and characterization of a cell line of human breast carcinoma origin. *Eur. J. Cancer.* 1979 May;15(5):659-70.

Lacroix M, Leclercq G. Relevance of breast cancer cell lines as models for breast tumours: an update. *Breast Cancer Res. Treat.* 2004 Feb;83(3):249-89.

Lacroix M. Persistent use of "false" cell lines. *Int. J. Cancer.* 2008 Jan 1;122(1):1-4.

Lacroix M. MDA-MB-435 cells are from melanoma, not from breast cancer. *CancerChemother.Pharmacol.* 2009 Feb;63(3):567.

Lasfargues EY, Ozzello L: Cultivation of human breast carcinomas. *J. Natl. Cancer Inst.* 1958 Dec;21(6):1131-47.

Lathrop AE, Loeb L. Further investigations on the origin of tumors in mice. III. On the part played by internal secretion in the spontaneous development of tumors. *J. Cancer Res.* 1916 Jan;1(1):1-19.

Leder H, Stewart TA. Transgenic non-human mammals. 1984. *Biotechnology.* 1992;24:556-63.

Levenson AS, Jordan VC. MCF-7: the first hormone-responsive breast cancer cell line. *Cancer Res.* 1997 Aug 1;57(15):3071-8.

Lieberman ME, Maurer RA, Gorski J. Estrogen control of prolactin synthesis in vitro. *Proc. Natl. Acad. Sci. U S A.* 1978 Dec;75(12):5946-9.

Li X, Lewis MT, Huang J, Gutierrez C, Osborne CK, Wu MF, Hilsenbeck SG, Pavlick A, Zhang X, Chamness GC, Wong H, Rosen J, Chang JC. Intrinsic resistance of tumorigenic breast cancer cells to chemotherapy. *J. Natl. Cancer Inst.* 2008 May 7;100(9):672-9.

Man S, Munoz R, Kerbel RS. On the development of models in mice of advanced visceral metastatic disease for anti-cancer drug testing. *Cancer Metastasis Rev.* 2007 Dec;26(3-4):737-47.

Russo J, Russo IH. Atlas and histologic classification of tumors of the rat mammary gland. *J. Mammary Gland Biol. Neoplasia.* 2000 Apr;5(2):187-200.

Shimkin MB. A. E. C. Lathrop (1868-1918): Mouse Woman of Granby. *Cancer Res.* 1975 Jun;35(6):1597-8.

Soule HD, Vazquez J, Long A, Albert S, Brennan M. A human cell line from a pleural effusion derived from a breast carcinoma. *J. Natl. Cancer Inst.* 1973 Nov;51(5):1409-16.

Stewart TA, Pattengale PK, Leder P. Spontaneous mammary adenocarcinomas in transgenic mice that carry and express MTV/myc fusion genes. *Cell.* 1984 Oct;38(3):627-37

Suntzeff V. Leo Loeb; 1869-1959. *Cancer Res.* 1960 Jul;20:972-3.

Thompson HJ, Singh M. Rat models of premalignant breast disease. *J. Mammary Gland Biol. Neoplas*ia. 2000 Oct;5(4):409-20.

Tomlinson GE, Chen TT, Stastny VA, Virmani AK, Spillman MA, Tonk V, Blum JL, Schneider NR, Wistuba II, Shay JW, Minna JD, Gazdar AF. Characterization of a breast cancer cell line derived from a germ-line BRCA1 mutation carrier. *Cancer Res.* 1998 Aug 1;58(15):3237-42.

Vargo-Gogola T, Rosen JM. Modelling breast cancer: one size does not fit all. *Nat. Rev. Cancer.* 2007 Sep;7(9):659-72.

Weigelt B, Bissell MJ. Unraveling the microenvironmental influences on the normal mammary gland and breast cancer. *Semin. Cancer Biol.* 2008 Oct;18(5):311-21.

Bibliography

Author unknown (translated by Veith, I.). *The yellow emperor's classic of internal medicine.* First edition. Berkeley, CA: University of California Press; 2002.

Barton-Burke., M, and Berg, D. *Cancer Chemotherapy: A Nursing Process Approach.* First edition. Boston, MA: Jones and Bartlett; 1996.

Bassett, LW., Jackson, V., Fu, K., and Fu, Y. *Diagnosis of Diseases of the Breast*, Second edition. Philadelphia PA : WB Saunders Company; 2005.

Batt, S. *Patient no more: the politics of breast cancer.* First edition. London (U.K.): Scarlet Press; 1994.

Beahrs, OH., Carr, DT., and Rubin, P. *Manual for Staging of Cancer.* First edition. Philadelphia PA: Lippincott; 1977.

Blake, MA., and Kalra, MK. *Imaging in Oncology* (Cancer Treatment and Research). First edition. New-York NY: Springer-Verlag; 2008.

Bland, KI., and Coeland, EM. *The breast: comprehensive management of benign and malignant diseases.* Second edition. Philadelphia PA: W.B. Saunders Company; 1998.

Bowcock, AM. *Breast Cancer: Molecular Genetics, Pathogenesis, and Therapeutics.* First edition. Totowa NJ: Humana Press; 1999.

Breasted, JH. *The Edwin Smith Surgical Papyrus.* First edition Chicago IL: University of Chicago Press; 1930.

Broca, P.P. *Traité des Tumeurs* (Vols. 1 and 2, in French). First edition. Paris (France): Asselin; 1866-1869.

Bynum, WF., and Porte, R. *Companion encyclopedia of the history of medicine.* First edition.New York NY: Routledge; 1993.

Cade, S. *Radium Treatment of Cancer.* First edition. London (U.K.): JandA Churchill; 1929.

Donegan, WL., and Spratt, JS. *Cancer of the breast*. Fifth edition. Philadelphia PA: WB Saunders Company; 2002.

Faguet, GB. *The war on cancer: an anatomy of failure, a blueprint for the future.*First edition. New-York NY: Springer-Verlag; 2005.

Grmek, MD. *Diseases in the Ancient Greek World*. First edition. Baltimore MD: The John Hopkins University Press; 1989.

Haagensen, CD. *Diseases of the breast*. First edition. Philadelphia PA : WB Saunders Company; 1971.

Harding, AS. *Milestones in Health and Medicine*. First edition. Phoenix AZ: Oryx Press; 2000.

Harris, JR., Lippman, ME., Osborne, CK., and Morrow, M. *Diseases of the breast*. Fourth edition. Philadelphia PA: Lippincott Williams and Wilkins; 2009.

Herodotus, and Rawlinson, G. *The Histories*. First edition. London (U.K.): J.M. Dent and Sons; 1992.

Hudis, CA., Norton, L., and Winchester, DJ. *Breast Cancer* (Atlas of Clinical Oncology). Second edition. Shelton CT: People's Medical Publishing House-USA; 2005.

Jatoi, I., Kaufmann, M., and Petit, JY. *Atlas of Breast Surgery*. First edition. New-York NY: Springer-Verlag;2006.

Kushner, R. *Breast cancer: a personal history and an investigative report*. First edition. San Diego CA: Harcourt Brace Jovanovich; 1975.

Lacroix, M. *Tumor Suppressor Genes in Breast Cancer*. First edition. Hauppauge NY: Nova Science Publishers; 2008.

Lacroix, M. M*olecular Therapy of Breast Cancer: Classicism Meets Modernity*. First edition. Hauppauge NY: Nova Science Publishers; 2009.

Lacroix, M. *MicroRNAs in Breast Cancer*. First edition. Hauppauge NY: Nova Science Publishers; 2010.

Lebert, H. Traité Pratique des Maladies Cancéreuses (in French). First edition. Paris (France): J.B. Bailliere ; 1851.

Lerner, BH. Breast *Cancer Wars : Hope, Fear, and the Pursuit of a Cure in Twentieth-Century America*. First edition.New York NY: Oxford University Press; 2001.

Mackay, J., Jemal, A., Lee, NC., and Parkin, DM. *The Cancer Atlas*. First edition. Atlanta GA: American Cancer Society; 2006.

McKinnell, RG., Parchment, RE., Perantoni, AO., Pierce, GB., and Damjanov, I. *The biological basis of cancer*. Second edition. Cambridge (U.K.): Cambridge University Press; 2006.

Nass, SJ., Henderson, IC., and Lashof, JC. *Mammography and Beyond: Developing Technologies for the Early Detection of Breast*. First edition. Washington DC: National Academy Press; 2001.

Nery, R. *Cancer: an Enigma in Biology and Society*. First edition. Philadelphia PA: Charles Pr Pub; 1986.

Nordenskiöld, E. *The history of biology: a survey.*First edition in English. New-York NY: Tudor Publishing and Co; 1946.

Nunn, TW. *On cancer of the breast*. First edition. London (U.K.): J. and A. Churchill; 1882.

O'Dowd, MJ., and Philipp, EE. *The History of Obstetrics and Gynaecology*. First edition.New York NY: Informa Healthcare; 2000.

Olson, JS. *Bathsheba's Breast: Women, Cancer, and History*. First edition. Baltimore MD: The Johns Hopkins University Press; 2005.

Pancoast, J. *A treatise of operative surgery*. First edition. Philadelphia PA: Carey and Hart; 1844.

Perry, MC. *The Chemotherapy Source Book*. Fourth edition. Philadelphia PA: Lippincott Williams and Wilkins; 2007.

Peters, WP., and Visscher, DW. *Breast Cancer*, Volume 2 (Advances in Oncobiology). First edition. Amsterdam (The Netherlands): Elsevier Science Publishers; 1998.

Raven, RW. *The theory and practice of oncology. Historical evolution and present principles*. First edition. Park Ridge NJ: The Parthenon Publishing Group; 1990.

Rawlinson, MC., and Lundeen, S. T*he voice of breast cancer in medicine and bioethics*. First edition. New-York NY: Springer-Verlag; 2006.

Rayter, Z., and Mansi, J. *Medical Therapy of Breast Cancer*. First edition. Cambridge (U.K.): Cambridge University Press; 2008.

Shaw De Paredes, E. *Atlas of Mammography*. Third edition. Philadelphia PA: Lippincott Williams and Wilkins; 2007.

Singletary, SE., Robb, GL., and Hortobagyi, GN. *Advanced therapy of breast disease*. Second edition. Hamilton (Canada): B.C. Decker; 2004.

Tavassoli, FA., and Devilee, P. World Health Organization: Tumours of the Breast and Female Genital Organs. First edition. Lyon (France): IARCPress-WHO; 2003.

UICC Committee on Clinical Stage Classification and Applied Statistics. Clinical Stage Classification and Presentation of Results, Malignant Tumors of the Breast and Larynx. First edition. Paris (France): International Union Against Cancer; 1958.

Velpeau, AA. Traité des maladies du sein et de la région mammaire (in French). First edition. Paris (France): Victor Masson; 1854.

Williams, P. *Breast Cancer*: Biography of an Illness. First edition. Toronto (Canada): BPS Books; 2008.

Yalom, M. *A History of the Breast*. First edition. New York NY: Ballantine Books; 1998.

Index

C

N

O

P

Q

R